# Social Work and Dementia

## Bradford Dementia Group Good Practice Guides

Originally under the editorship of Professor Tom Kitwood, and reflecting his commitment to the person-centred approach to dementia, this series draws on both experience in practice and the latest research in the fields of dementia and dementia care. It provides a set of accessible, jargon-free good practice guides for the carers of people with dementia.

**Training and Development for Dementia Care Workers**
*Anthea Innes*
ISBN 1 85302 761 8
*Bradford Dementia Group Good Practice Guides*

**Drug Treatments and Dementia**
*Stephen Hopker*
ISBN 1 85302 760 X
*Bradford Dementia Group Good Practice Guides*

**The Pool Activity Level (PAL) Instrument**
A Practical Resource for Carers of People with Dementia
*Jackie Pool*
ISBN 1 85302 813 4
*Bradford Dementia Group Good Practice Guides*

*of related interest*

**Including the Person with Dementia in Designing and Delivering Care**
'I Need to Be Me!'
*Elizabeth Barnett*
ISBN 1 85302 740 5

**Hearing the Voice of People with Dementia**
Opportunities and Obstacles
*Malcolm Goldsmith*
ISBN 1 85302 406 6

**Confused Professionals**
The Social Construction of Dementia
*Nancy H. Harding and Colin Palfrey*
ISBN 1 85302 257 8

**Understanding Dementia**
The Man with the Worried Eyes
*Richard Cheston and Michael Bender*
ISBN 1 85302 479 1

Bradford Dementia Group Good Practice Guides

# Social Work and Dementia
## Good Practice and Care Management

Margaret Anne Tibbs

Foreword by Murna Downs

Jessica Kingsley Publishers
London and Philadelphia

First published in the United Kingdom in 2001 by
Jessica Kingsley Publishers Ltd
116 Pentonville Road, London
N1 9JB, England
and
325 Chestnut Street,
Philadelphia, PA 19106, USA.

*www.jkp.com*

**Library of Congress Cataloging in Publication Data**
A CIP catalog record for this book is available from the Library of Congress

**British Library Cataloguing in Publication Data**
A CIP catalogue record for this book is available from the British Library

ISBN 1 85302 904 1

Printed and Bound in Great Britain by
Athenaeum Press, Gateshead, Tyne and Wear

# Contents

Acknowledgements                                    6

Dedication                                          7

A note on language                                  8

Foreword by Murna Downs                             9

1. Introduction                                    11

2. The Journey Through Care                        19

3. The Historical and Legal Context                39

4. Good Practice in Social Work with
   People with Dementia and Their Carers           68

5. The Emotional and Social World of
   the Person with Dementia                        96

6. Cultural Difference                            123

7. The Road Ahead – Directions for the Future     141

   Appendix I A Short Guide for the Management
   of Finances for a Person with Dementia         162

   Appendix II Some Useful Contacts for
   Social Workers                                 166

   References                                     171

   Index                                          173

# Acknowledgements

I would like to thank the late Professor Tom Kitwood who suggested that I should write this book, encouraged me, gave me his valuable time and acted as my editor. I would also like to thank Professor Neil Small of the School of Health Studies at the University of Bradford and Anthea Innes and Errollyn Bruce of the Bradford Dementia Group at the University for reading the manuscript. Above all I must thank Professor Murna Downs of the University of Bradford who took over the editorial role after the death of Tom Kitwood, devoting much time and effort to the project.

I would also like to thank the social workers of the North Bedfordshire Department of Social and Community Care with whom I worked for ten years. Specifically I am indebted to those who worked with me in the Pathfinder Team in Bedford. They were my colleagues during the time that we developed the community mental health team for older people in the area. Sian McDonagh-McCloskey, Rebecca Chowdhury, Linda Gibbs and Dr. Julia Cream of the Alzheimer's Society have also given me assistance recently for which I am grateful.

This book is the result of my experiences and my reflections on those experiences during the years I spent working in social services in North Bedfordshire.

*To John*

# A note on language

Language has changed and keeps changing in social work. I have, therefore, decided to use the following terms:

**social workers**   rather than 'care manager' or 'care organizer.' Social services departments are using different terms at different times to describe the role. I feel that 'social worker' is understood by us all.

**client**   I have sometimes used this word instead of 'service user' or 'customer'. But I prefer, where possible, to use the person-centred convention of using the phrase 'person with dementia'.

**family**   in an attempt to use inclusive language I have substituted 'partner' for 'spouse'. However, I have retained 'family' as this can include many different types of structure.

**social services**   these departments now have many different titles as their function has changed, depending on local conditions. I have chosen, for the sake of clarity, to retain the term 'social services', which is familiar.

# Foreword

Social work and dementia care have undergone dramatic changes in the last 10 years. *Social Work and Dementia* charts these developments and articulates a contemporary best practice for social work in this area. The field of dementia used to be concerned with depicting the extent of dysfunction and deficit in the person with dementia and with documenting the degree of burden, stress and burnout experienced by their carers. *Social Work and Dementia* charts our current thinking which stresses the potential for improving quality of life for both people with dementia and their families. It articulates a social work practice that reflects this new culture in dementia care. More importantly it confronts the challenges and dilemmas that a person-centred approach raises for social work practice. *Social Work and Dementia* offers useful suggestions for addressing the difficulties associated with assessment and referral to services that have therapeutic potential for people with dementia and their families. The book combines a sound basis in day-to-day social work practice within the context of theoretical and practice developments alongside legislative and policy changes.

*Murna Downs*
*Professor in Dementia Studies*
*Bradford Dementia Group*
*University of Bradford*

# CHAPTER ONE

# Introduction

This book aims to fill a significant gap in the literature about social care for people with dementia. This gap is related to social work and dementia.

This is a time of great change in the field of social work and in the field of dementia. Because the context in which social work operates is changing and because we now have a different view of dementia, it seems to be a good time to take a fresh look at the role of the social worker in this field.

The context in which social work operates has changed significantly in some respects. There can be no doubt that the care of people with dementia is now firmly on the national agenda. The number of people with dementia is approaching one million. Alzheimer's Society – Information Section (2000). Most of the responsibility of caring for this very large number of people with dementia still falls on families. It is important to remember that, at any one time, 80 per cent of people with dementia are living at home in the community (*ibid.*).

The role of the social worker whose job is based within the community, therefore, is of key importance as we consider the best ways to meet the changing needs of the person with dementia and those who care for them. Major reform of the National Health Service is underway, with the government announcing plans to create what is beginning to be referred to as a 'new NHS' which will be more effective in meeting the increasing health needs and the higher expectations of an ageing population. The government is strongly emphasizing the need to provide a seamless service of health care between community and hospital, and the phrase 'joined up' care services has become popular. But there is an admission, in spite of the rhetoric of the past decade, that this objective has not yet been achieved.

A document entitled *Modernising Health and Social Services: National Priorities Guidance 1999/00–2001/02* (Department of Health 1998) outlines a three-year plan to which all parts of the NHS and social services will be expected to contribute. Crucially, it treats the health and social care system as one. Social services departments are now, according to the government, to be regarded as part of the new NHS, and strong messages are coming from central government that the only way to meet the nation's health care needs is for both halves of the 'health care system' to work together in a way which has not yet been achieved. 'A drive to tackle inequality, break down barriers, improve standards and speed up services requires a new approach for health and social services' Department of Health (1998, p.19).

## A TIME OF CHANGE

These statements from central and local government are to be welcomed, but the real challenge will be in turning such theory into practice, such rhetoric into reality.

The public is becoming aware that people over seventy-five form a high percentage of the patients who occupy much needed acute hospital beds after their need for acute hospital care has passed. They are remaining in hospital because they are not well enough to return home to live independently without additional social care, which is provided through social services. The government is now saying that the solution to this problem is to provide what it refers to as 'intermediate care' for this group of people. Recognition must now be given to the fact that people with dementia constitute a significant subgroup of those people who need this 'intermediate' type of care. The National Service Framework for Older People is a welcome addition to government guidance about how best to meet the health needs of our ageing population (2001).

The recent Audit Commission report *Forget Me Not Mental Health Services for Older People* (Audit Commission 2000) quoted some very telling statistical facts:

- the number of people over 65 is predicted to rise by 10 per cent in the next 10 years

- the greatest increase will be among those over 80

- one-quarter of those over 85 develop dementia

- one-third of these people (the 25% of people over 85 who develop dementia) need constant care or supervision.

Many people who are caring for people with dementia are elderly themselves. Levin, Moriarty and Gorbach found in their study of 530 carers of people with dementia that 57 per cent of the subjects were husbands or wives. Two-thirds of the sample were aged over 65, the oldest member being aged 92 (Levin, *et al.*1994, p.14).

More recently, in 1998, a government survey of 'informal' carers found that they were most likely to be aged between 45 and 64. Over half of all carers look after someone aged over 75, and two out of ten carers are caring for a spouse (Office for National Statistics 1998).

As well as these changes in the context of the health and social care environment, we now know much more about dementia than ever before. Our understanding about the way the brain works and our medical knowledge about dementia are greater than ever before. But we are no longer content to describe dementia in terms of the standard framework or paradigm, which viewed it as an irreversible, progressive, degenerative neurological condition leading inevitably to the death of brain cells and the loss of the person (through catastrophic changes in the brain).

This paradigm was described by Tom Kitwood as 'a simple linear idea, along the lines of a billiard cue setting one ball in motion, and this colliding into another, causing it to move as well, and so on' (Kitwood 1997, p.35). It implies that once a person has developed dementia, their story will inevitably be one of decay, decline and despair. This view is sometimes referred to as the 'disaster view of dementia'.

The standard paradigm has proved to be inadequate, either to explain the experience of dementia or, indeed, to help people who develop it to achieve their optimum state of well-being.

Tom Kitwood, who was so influential through his writing in changing this standard paradigm and reframing a more optimistic alternative, wrote:

> After a century and more of research into dementia, mainly within the standard paradigm, we have heard just about all that might be cause for dismay. As we now reframe the whole field, and give much greater weight to personal and interpersonal considerations, most of what follows will be good news. We will discover much more about how to enable people who have dementia to fare well, without having to wait for magic bullets or technical fixes. (Kitwood 1997, p.6)

It was Kitwood who coined the phrase 'new culture' of dementia care and described it in the following terms:

> The old culture is one of alienation and estrangement. Through it we are distanced from our fellow human beings, deprived of our insight, cut off from our own vitality. The old culture is one of domination, technique, evasion and buck-passing. To enter the new culture is like coming home. We can now draw close to other human beings, accepting all that we genuinely share. We can recover confidence in our power to know, to discover, to give, to create, to love. And

this homecoming is a cause for joy and celebration. (Kitwood and Benson 1995, p.11)

This idea is revolutionary in terms of the way we care for people with dementia. We now know that the experience of dementia means different things to different people. We know from our personal experience when our emotional world is diminished that emotional needs can be experienced as overwhelmingly powerful. Above all we have learned that dementia must be placed within the context of the personality, the relationships the person is having, the life history and the physical health of the person. This means that we can no longer dismiss all the behaviours of disruption and protest shown by people with dementia as simply being symptomatic of a failing brain which no longer functions properly. We now realize that we must try to understand these behaviours in order to learn what the person is trying to communicate through them to the world around.

The new culture of dementia care has developed rapidly from the mid-1990s, as professionals in the field have taken on board the new ideas and tried to transform them into better care practice in the light of this new understanding. The Dementia Services Development Centres and the *Journal of Dementia Care* are making significant contributions to this great common endeavour. The decision made by the Alzheimer's Society and Alzheimer Scotland – Action on Dementia, to focus on the needs of the person with dementia as well as the needs of those who care for them (the original focus of these great voluntary societies), has also been extremely significant. This is, indeed, a time of rapid and important change within the field.

Social workers play a pivotal role in the lives of people with dementia and their families and others who care for them. Their intervention at various key points in the dementia journey is crucial. Significantly, a large percentage of older people who still fall within the high priority group, as defined under current social services eligibility criteria, are people with dementia.

This pivotal role is not generally recognized. Perhaps it is not fully recognized by the profession. However, the fact remains that for every individual who approaches health or social services for assistance, the process has to start with an assessment of need. If public money is to be spent, this assessment must be carried out by a local authority social worker. The decisions which social workers make, and their ability to act as advocates for the individuals concerned, are crucial to the best outcomes for the person with dementia.

Skilful assessment of the situation and construction of the care package is vital. So is the ability to make frequent adaptations as the situation changes. The ability of the social worker to empathize with the bewilderment and loss felt by the person with dementia, and by those who are caring for them, is also crucial. So is their ability to help individuals to work through the pain they are feeling. Most importantly, good social work practice can dramatically increase the well-being of the person with dementia and of those who care for them.

If the social worker does not possess sufficient skill or experience, a minor problem may develop into a major crisis. In a worst-case scenario a person with dementia may be admitted prematurely to an acute hospital, and go from there to a long-term place in a residential or nursing home. Conversely, skilful case management may help the family to support the person in their own home for a much longer period of time. It can avert a crisis admission to hospital and thus prevent the blocking of a precious, acute hospital bed.

There is little evidence that social workers are given the attention they need and deserve within the growing body of literature and research about social care for people with dementia. Much is now written by and for nurses, occupational therapists, and psychologists, and by providers of social care, but there is a marked absence of practice-based books for social workers working in this field. A notable exception, of course, is the key text *Dementia – New Skills for Social Workers* (Chapman and

Marshall 1993), although it was published before the National Health Service and Community Care Act reforms had taken full effect.

The reason for this lack of emphasis on good dementia social-work practice may partly be that when the NHS and Community Care Act (1990) created the purchaser–provider split in social services in 1993, social workers found themselves on the purchaser side of the great divide. The considerable expertise that has been developed in social care and dementia since 1993 has been developed on the provider side of social care. Social workers have, in effect, become isolated from the growing body of knowledge which is developing in the field of dementia care, and specialist social-work expertise in the field is still generally lacking. Training for social workers in assessment and care planning for people with dementia still fails to be given a high priority within the profession, although people with dementia make up a significant proportion of the cases being assessed by social workers who work with older people.

Chapter Two of this book describes the role of the social worker in helping people with dementia and their carers as they move through the social care system. In order to place our current situation in context, Chapter Three goes on to examine the key legislative policy initiatives within which social-work services have developed, and some of the challenges which face social workers as a result. Social work and care management with people who have dementia is discussed in Chapter Four, with an emphasis on examining the specialist skills which are needed when working in this field. In Chapter Five the particular challenges facing social workers who are trying to apply the principles of person-centred care within care management, are explored. Chapter Six highlights the need to pay attention to cultural difference in the experience of and response to dementia. In Chapter Seven some future trends in government policy are discussed, and a suggested model for a social-work service for people with dementia is described. A useful appendix

(1) on specialist financial and legal expertise, which is needed by the social worker in this field, is provided at the end.

The gap between theory and practice is a recurring theme within the book. In 1993 the NHS and Community Care Act stated that the emphasis of all social work assessments must change from being service-led to being needs-led. The pressures on local authority spending and the ongoing budgetary constraints since 1993 have meant that it has not yet been possible in many areas to implement this change. Shortage of resources seems to be used as a justification for the continued culture of paternalism, which has historically existed within local authority social services departments and prevents the empowerment of the consumer. The goal of making needs-led assessments still proves elusive. This remains as a challenge to all social workers. It is particularly difficult for social workers who are working with adults who have impaired insight and judgement and are unable to tell their social worker what they feel they need for themselves.

It is my belief that people with dementia have specialized needs and that those needs will best be met by social workers who possess specialist skills and knowledge acquired through education and training as well as experience. It is my hope that this book will help social workers to improve their own practice and make their own unique contribution to the growing body of knowledge and skills in the field of dementia care.

# CHAPTER TWO

# The Journey Through Care

## INTRODUCTION

The purpose of this chapter is to outline the role of social work in helping with individuals' and families' experience of living with dementia, from the earliest signs that something is wrong to coming to terms with the death of the person they have been caring for.

It is common to think of living with dementia as a journey. As a journey, however, living with dementia may have no clear starting point and its path is often unpredictable. People find themselves initially following a track, which may be almost unseen. Then the track turns into a clear pathway, which begins to lead them through the system of social and medical support. In general terms this path follows the trajectory of the process of the dementia.

However, because the experience of dementia means different things to different people and has a different impact upon their carers, this path does not follow a straight and smooth course. If one imagines the path, one might expect that it would start at the top of a hill and continue downwards in a way which is clearly visible to an observer standing at the top. But the matter is not so straightforward. The path twists and turns, with unexpected plunges down the hillside followed by relatively smooth plateaux. A succession of hairpin bends may be followed by the occasional long, straight passage which is easy for the observer to see.

## PREDICTABLE TIMES WHEN THERE MAY BE AN INTERFACE WITH SOCIAL WORK

Once the person has embarked on the path into dementia we can observe another common phenomenon. We know from casework experience that there are specific points at which we can predict that additional support will be needed. The availability of the right kind of support will determine whether one of these points of significant change develops into a crisis or not.

From the point of view of the person with dementia and those who are caring for them, the journey is a process of living with dementia, and this is how the process may be described from a person-centred perspective. However, in terms of the social-work task, which still remains firmly orientated in problem-solving and in the provision of services, the journey may be better described through the various points (outlined below) where contact is made with the services which are available. The social worker should remember that these two perspectives co-exist with each other. The contact with social services may occupy a brief period in what is, for many people, a journey which lasts for several years.

### From first suspicions that something is wrong to diagnosis

Many families experience a period of stress and uncertainty before the diagnosis of dementia is made. Alzheimer's disease, in particular, which is the most common cause of dementia, starts insidiously so that it is often only those who know the person intimately who realise that something is wrong. Many GPs have been notoriously ineffective in providing the kind of support which their patients need at this point. And it has long been recognised by workers in the field that the period before and immediately after diagnosis is often very difficult for all concerned. The fact that the person with dementia has not usually been told their own diagnosis adds to the uncertainty and fear. Experience would suggest that for many people a close emotional relationship between the person with dementia and the carer means that changes in that relationship caused by the dementia, or by the news that the person has dementia, are likely to cause feelings of loss and anxiety. This is often very marked in the case of couples who have shared their lives for many decades.

In the case of elderly couples, the changes in the relationship which living with impairment brings can be very hard to handle, because the loss of physical health and strength which commonly occurs over the age of sixty-five undermines resilience. Long-established mechanisms for coping with distress often prove to be inadequate in this situation. The co-dependency which often exists between couples who have lived together for many years makes it hard for them to cope with the losses which often accompany dementia. Ignorance and fear about dementia is widespread in the population as a whole, and people simply do not know what to expect when they are told that they, or their partner, is suffering from dementia.

However, it may be equally devastating for other family members. Adult children, particularly daughters, often seem to find acceptance of such a diagnosis very traumatic – coinciding, as it often does, with other stressful events in their own lives, such as the menopause or children leaving home. In my own experience it is also not at all unusual for people in their sixties and seventies to be acting as primary carers for a parent in their nineties. At a time when people might reasonably expect to be looked after themselves, they can find that they are caring for a parent who is entirely dependent on them.

The failure of many GPs to offer adequate support at this time is well documented. The *Forget Me Not* report (Audit Commission 2000) referred to above found, for instance, that one-half of the carers surveyed were not told by their GP what the problem was, or how dementia was likely to affect their relative in the future. Written information for carers was readily available in only four out of the twelve areas surveyed by the Audit Commission. By the time that families reach the social worker, they may have had a period of weeks, months or even years of increasingly desperate attempts to find out what is wrong with the person and to obtain help.

Social workers have been aware for some time that carers are often very anxious throughout the whole period which starts when they first perceive that something is wrong with their person, and lasts through the making of the diagnosis to the full acceptance of what that diagnosis means. But, until recently, little attention has been paid to the feelings and wishes of the person with dementia at the time of diagnosis. General practitioners have also been notoriously reluctant to make a definite diagnosis. An attitude of professional nihilism in the face of the absence of effective therapies has often led to GPs doing nothing at this point. The systems reflect the fact that the person with dementia is not, at present, truly involved in the process. This is one of several areas in dementia care in the community where we have not yet got it right.

The social worker should make every effort to persuade the carer to make contact with a local carers' support group if there is one as soon after diagnosis as possible. If the carer is resistant at that time, as many people are, the social worker should continue to remind them about the existence of support groups at intervals during the course of the dementia. Their needs will change as the situation changes.

It is not always appreciated by professionals who lack specific expertise in dementia that the task of caring for somebody 24 hours a day, 365 days a year can deprive the carer of their normal social life, not to mention all the other losses which are easier to identify. Life tends to shrink for the person with dementia and for their carer, and their friends begin to drift away. It becomes harder and harder for people in this situation to socialize. By referring people to a self-help organization where a social life can be re-created, the social worker is making a very important contribution to the well-being of the carer and the person with dementia.

Younger people with dementia have begun to be seen as a group in their own right, with care needs which differ from those of very elderly people. As differential diagnosis improves, people with, for example, frontal lobe dementia and Pick's disease (which usually affect people under sixty-five), are now identified as distinct groups. This earlier diagnosis means that more people are coming 'into the system' at a point when they still have insight into their condition. They may have clear ideas about what type of care they require and will certainly be experiencing strong emotions as they come to terms with their diagnosis.

The question of whether or not to share the diagnosis with the person with dementia is now hotly discussed in professional dementia circles. More people are now being told their diagnosis. It is possible to infer this from referrals to the Alzheimer's Society national helpline. In 1997 there were 77 people who referred themselves to the Alzheimer's Society through the national helpline, following diagnosis. In 1998 this figure had almost doubled to 126 (Alzheimer's Society – Information Section, 2000).

## Community care

### Day care

It seems that day care – usually the first card in the pack of care services to be offered – is accepted without too much difficulty by carers. They find it acceptable and are often greatly relieved to find that they have a break of a few hours a day from the task of caring. As Levin *et al.* found in their survey, 'the majority of carers with day care valued the regular, reliable weekly breaks it afforded them. Importantly, most of these carers thought that day care also benefited their relatives' (Levin *et al.*1994, p.73).

People with dementia, however, do not always find it so acceptable. They may never have been 'joiners' and do not react favourably to the idea of participating in group activities with other people whom they do not know. In this case it is not a useful form of respite. However, for many people, after a careful introduction, it becomes a thoroughly enjoyable experience.

New friendships are made with others who attend, and with staff. A break from being cared for at home by an increasingly stressed partner can become as acceptable to the person with dementia as it is to their carer, as it allows them to spend several hours in an environment which is tailor-made to their needs and in which they do not feel a failure. The well-being of the person can be clearly improved. However, it is important to be honest about what is on offer and what day care entails, so that both parties understand its benefits and its limitations.

Twenty-three per cent of people with dementia live alone (Alzheimer's Society – Information Section, 2000), but for them the improvement in their quality of life during the few hours they spend in company at the day centre could highlight the loneliness and isolation of their existence. This should be taken into account when the care package is being set up. After the busy hours spent at the day centre, the next human to be seen by the person may be a home carer who calls the next morning for half an hour to check that s/he is all right. The life led by many people with dementia living alone is shockingly empty of human company. Respite day care may work extremely well for them, alleviating their loneliness for a period of time, but it may also exacerbate the loneliness of the rest of their lives. Respite is a double-edged sword.

The majority of people with dementia, however, are living with others, and the significant thing is that they will return home to their carers at the end of the day. After an initial careful period of introduction, day care can become an acceptable form of support to both parties.

## Home care

The more traditional type of homecare is also offered in many areas of the country, where help is given to the person to get up in the morning and to go to bed at night, and to ensure that they eat at least one hot meal a day. Again, the service is offered to people who live alone as well as to those who live with carers. In this type of service, however, the home carer is more likely to perform the tasks, including personal care, for the person.

This service helps the carer and ensures that the person is physically cared for within their own home, but the service – which is usually offered by private home care agencies – does not allow for sufficient time to be spent with the person to encourage independence. It does not offer a person-centred approach to care.

In some areas schemes exist which offer relief or respite care within the person's own home. A home careworker comes into the home to look after the person for a few hours at a time, enabling the carer to take a break. Depending on different factors, such as the weather and the physical health of the person, they may either take them out to the shops or for outings to local places, or they may initiate activities which the person enjoys at home. This type of respite care is offered where the person with dementia is living alone or where there is a resident carer. In the latter case the carer is then free to go out on their own or to carry out household tasks which otherwise do not get done. Care is taken to match the careworker(s) with the person with dementia so that friendships may be developed. This type of person-centred service is particularly useful in helping people with dementia to maintain their own skills, as well as in rebuilding their self-esteem.

## Residential respite care

For many people with dementia and for their carers the time will come when the carer can no longer provide supervision and support for twenty-four hours a day without a break. Residential respite care appears to be the obvious solution. The professionals offering this service tend to assume, if they are not well trained in dementia care, that everybody is going to be relieved and grateful when this service is offered. This is not so. Many carers will absolutely refuse to take this step until they are almost at the point of complete physical and emotional exhaustion.

There are many reasons for this. Some people refuse for financial reasons. The person requesting this service is financially assessed and means testing is applied. If the carer does not qualify for any financial assistance from the local authority, the full cost may be considerable. Some carers simply believe that nobody can look after the person as well as they can. Their fear of low-quality service may or may not be well founded. Almost certainly the staffing ratios in residential care homes mean that people will not receive nearly as much one-to-one attention as they do at home.

However, if the carer and the person with dementia are carefully prepared regarding what to expect, and the carer advised and informed beforehand about how best to handle the situation, the residential respite service can be extremely beneficial. It needs to be offered as flexibly as possible. The carer should be able to have a break of two or three nights or maybe two or three weeks.

The social worker needs to be aware that it is the carer who really benefits from respite care in the short term. (Levin *et al.*1994). It appears to enable the person with dementia to remain at home longer because it gives the carer a rest. Arguably this is what the person with dementia and the carer both want, and it is probably of benefit in the long run.

Certainly government policy is based on the assumption that this is so. In the document which sets out The National Strategy for Carers entitled *Caring about Carers*, Point 10 states:

> we that caring is founded on close relationships. The caring role grows out of the relationship and is one which most carers undertake from choice. Our objective is, therefore, focused on enabling those who choose to care, and those whose care is wanted by another person, to do so without detriment to the carer's inclusion in society and to their health. Our aim is to help support people who choose to be carers. (Audit Commission 1998, p.13)

The carer, however, may not particularly enjoy sending the person to respite care in the short term, at least initially.

The social worker should be aware, and should warn the carer, that in some cases the person will return home more confused after a respite short stay. Eleven per cent of carers in Levin *et al.* study reported that the person they cared for had deteriorated after the short stay, with increased confusion being the problem most often reported (Levin *et al.* 1994, p.112).

Social workers should be aware of the dangers in a situation where the carer begins to ask for so much respite that the person with dementia feels like an unwanted parcel. This kind of situation – where the person is already having day care twice a week and is then being taken to respite care for one week in three – gives a clear message: the carer is having difficulty coping. If that situation arises – and it does quite frequently – the carer needs help from the social worker to ask themselves why they are feeling like this and whose needs they are actually meeting? They need to be helped to acknowledge that there is no shame or blame if they feel that they cannot continue to care at home. When care is needed for twenty-four hours a day the time has probably come for the carer to hand over to a residential care home.

## Acute hospital care

Social workers often get involved with people with dementia at their time of admission to or discharge from hospital.

### Admission

There is clearly great pressure on acute hospital beds within the NHS at present and GPs often have a great struggle to find a bed for their older patients. The admission means that a very old person, who is already confused and is now acutely ill or injured, is admitted into a confusing and frightening situation – an acute hospital. Because they react to this with fear and distress they are often given sedation in order that their behaviour should not disrupt the hospital ward. Systems for liaison with the primary care team need to be greatly strengthened. It is clear that hospital admission can be a very significant point of deterioration for some people.

### Assessment

The assessment of need is then made, based upon the evidence of the person's behaviour in that strange situation. The people making the assessment, who may be meeting the person for the first time, react to him or her as they see them. But this is not an accurate picture. Many people are currently assessed as needing twenty-four-hour nursing or residential care, and discharged to what is felt to be an appropriate place, although with proper care they could regain their skills.

Specialist residential homes for people with dementia accommodate many people who were assessed in hospital as being agitated, aggressive, incontinent, refusing to eat, and needing the help of two nurses to walk. At the review meeting some weeks later the social worker may meet a resident who is fully mobile, only needs help and supervision to remain continent, and eats well, but really does not want to be in residential care. However, in my experience, it is very rare for them to succeed in returning home.

The window of opportunity for very elderly people to regain their independence is very small. People lose mobility, and motivation to live independently, at a speed which is frightening to watch. This means that they will become fully dependent very quickly if their independence is taken away from them too soon. It is clear that the assessment made in hospital at this pivotal point is in urgent need of reform.

## Discharge

Many of those who are caught in the struggle between the NHS and social services over who should pay for their care are people with dementia. Many people who are currently known colloquially and pejoratively as 'bed blockers' in acute beds in general hospitals belong to the group with whom we are concerned in this book.

Unlike their peers, who are physically frail but mentally capable, it is often impossible to discharge them from hospital and back into the community without an adequate care package because they are just too vulnerable. They become, as we all know, a bone of contention, caught between the hospital consultant who wants his bed free, the hard-pressed nursing staff caring for physically seriously ill patients, the social worker who is unable to complete an accurate assessment of need, the social services budget holder who does not have enough funding to pay for a long-term care place, and the family. Most hospitals are keen to achieve discharge as quickly as possible. Harassed acute hospital staff seem unable to give confused elderly patients the care they need. Stories from equally harassed relatives of people with dementia, who experience hospital care as neglectful and uninformed, have become commonplace. It may be significant that the situation has deteriorated since the closure of the cottage hospitals, which used to look after these people until proper arrangements could be made. A government initiative on the expansion of 'intermediate care' is very welcome. This follows the publication of the National Beds Inquiry (Department of Health 2000), which showed, according to Alan Milburn MP, Secretary of State for Health, that

> two-thirds of hospital beds are occupied by people aged 65 or over. It implies a radically different approach to the management of care in the NHS. That care has traditionally been about dealing with life's incidents – heart attacks and broken bones. Now an ageing population and increasing chronic disease means NHS care has also to be about dealing with life's experiences – getting older and becoming frailer. (p.21)

At a Kings Fund seminar the Secretary of State said that

> services for older people need to be reshaped. They should include a new set of intermediate care services specifically designed around the needs of older people for a period of rehabilitation and recovery, 'building a bridge between home and hospital'. (Kings Fund 2000)

It is hoped that health care planners will take into account the fact that a high proportion of this group consists of people with dementia. Hospital staff will need additional training in dementia if they are to offer the appropriate type of care.

In my experience, there is clear evidence to indicate that people with dementia often deteriorate rapidly after a hospital admission. This often leads to a second move, usually to a nursing home. This could be avoided if hospital staff had a better understanding of the needs of people with dementia, and the reasons why they behave as they do. If careful planning for discharge back to the residential home was started very soon after the surgery or acute medical treatment, many more people could return to the place they now regard as home.

Decisions which will affect someone's future life chances are in many cases based on an inadequate assessment of the person.

The social worker who attends hospital case conferences often feels like a nut being squeezed in a nutcracker because of the conflicting demands placed upon him/her. It is a very stressful position to be in – one of those in which work with people with dementia brings additional stress in comparison to work with people of the same age who are physically frail but mentally intact. The fact that the patient in hospital is able neither to tell others how they feel, nor to explain what they want to happen with respect to their future care, adds an extra dimension of uncertainty to the situation.

## When the decision is made to place a relative in a long-term residential or nursing home

This brings me to the next meeting-point between the social worker and the person with dementia in the journey through care. The decision to move someone into long-term care is rarely made without distress for those who are close to them. A small group of people with dementia are anxious to leave the responsibility of running their own lives and hand it over to someone else. There is a minority of individuals who feel lonely and isolated and who are aware that they can no longer manage on their own. However, in most cases, both those with dementia and their carers need a lot of help to come to the point of accepting the move to long-term care.

Popular language does not help. People still talk about 'putting someone away'. When a family can no longer care for an old person it is often seen as a failure of love – both by the person concerned and by those who care for them. Elderly parents still extract promises from their children that they will never let them be 'put away in a home', so that when this becomes inevitable the children or spouse feel guilty and the person feels rejected. Even in situations where the process of caring has brought the carer to the edge of physical and/or emotional collapse, the decision is very hard to make. For most people the decision is taken as a result of a crisis, e.g. deterioration in the physical health of the main carer, or a marked increase in the care needs of the person with dementia. Some families seem to 'manufacture' crises in order to give themselves permission to make this decision. Others need permission from a professional in order to do so.

The role of the social worker is to be aware of, and able to respond to, the emotions which are likely to be present at this stage of the older person's life. The person concerned may feel strong emotions – anxiety bordering on panic, a sense of rejection or even abandonment by the family, anger that this decision has been made, and/or an overwhelming sense of loss. The carer(s) may feel an initial sense of euphoric relief – but in many cases this is short-lived. They will almost certainly feel guilt. They may well express anxiety about whether the residential/nursing home will be able to provide such good care as they have done, by which they probably mean the amount of one-to-one attention which the person will receive. The answer to that question is – of course – that it will not. No home will be able to provide one-to-one attention twenty-four hours a day. The care staff will not be familiar, at least in most care settings, with all the personal likes and dislikes, routines and emotional needs of the new resident. However, the fact that staff members are not as emotionally involved with the person can be an advantage. Stress between the person who is caring and the person who is cared for may have reached a high level within the family home.

Some people who have spent most of each day alone at home seem to take on a new lease of life when they move to long-term care. Their loneliness is alleviated by the presence of other people and they thrive in the sociable atmosphere of group living. However, it should also be remembered that moving an older person with dementia from his or her own home is a high-risk strategy. Other professionals may need reminding of this fact when they are pressing that 'Mrs. So and So should be put in a home immediately because she is not safe at home'.

People often have falls in unfamiliar surroundings. They often die within a few weeks of a move to a new home. Social workers who work in this field know this.

## The difficulty of making the decision

This creates a potent emotional mix. The social worker must be able to work sensitively and skilfully with all the family at this time. It is, of course, much easier for everyone when the person has become accustomed to residential care following regular respite care, and when the carer has become accustomed to this kind of separation. The best possible solution is when a residential place becomes available in the home where respite care has been given. (Unfortunately, the pressures on the social care system are such that it is luck rather than anything else when the vacancy occurs in the right home at the right time.)

The situation is made more difficult for everyone because the person with dementia is not able to give – and remember that they have given – 'informed consent' to the decision. The loss of insight which accompanies dementia makes this decision very difficult. Often the person will believe quite sincerely that they can manage perfectly well on their own, and appeals to reason will inevitably fall on deaf ears.

It is always right to be honest with the person about the decision – but it is the task of the family to tell their relative. The social worker would only do this if there were no family. The family was a family before this decision had to be made, and will continue to be a family afterwards. They must work out a way of relating to each other which will survive this difficult period. Residential care staff are faced with a very difficult task if the person has not been told the truth – if they have agreed to come for a short visit, and then find that they are not going home. This is very cruel to the person with dementia. It is also cruel to tell them starkly that they are never going home again. The information is probably best given in stages, in a very sensitive manner.

## The Alzheimer's self-help movement

Carers need help and support at the point where the person they have been caring for goes into long-term care. The caring task may have taken over their life to such a degree that the rest of life seems to have disappeared. Hobbies have been abandoned, friends have disappeared, and social contacts have vanished. Unfortunately the statutory system is not able to offer support once the person with dementia has died. The loving support offered by other carers, who have been through the same experience themselves, is probably the best form of help anyway. Social workers should be sure to have contact numbers and addresses for local carers' support groups and contacts to offer their carer clients at this point.

Self-help carers' groups are currently supporting carers in many different countries throughout the world, using the self-help model, supported by professional training and expertise. It is true to say that sometimes, without their contribution, the social care infrastructure would collapse entirely. The carers groups are run largely by ex-carers. In the case of the Alzheimer's Society the network is supported in turn by a highly professional infrastructure, run from the national office in London with regional offices throughout England, Wales and Northern Ireland. Alzheimer Scotland – a sister organization – does the same job in Scotland. A directory of local branches and support groups can be obtained from the national offices.

Most people can be supported adequately through this network. It is important to put people in touch with the Alzheimer's Society or Alzheimer Scotland – Action on Dementia, if social workers are unable to offer support because the individual does not meet the eligibility criteria set by the local authority. The expertise they offer is invaluable in many ways.

The Alzheimer's movement is now a powerful pressure group for better care, more research and improved services throughout the world. The national Alzheimer's associations in Europe are in an affiliation called Alzheimer Europe, and all countries with associations belong to an organization called Alzheimer's Disease International, which holds an annual conference in a different country every year. Every year more countries join. Currently the fastest growing number of people with dementia is in the developing world, for example, in India and South America, where populations are beginning to age rapidly. As life expectancy increases, so does the prevalence of dementia.

## Helping people to settle in to long-term care

People have a right to the feelings they experience, and the settling-in process will be the better if they are allowed and encouraged to express their feelings of loss, betrayal, abandonment, etc. If people are furious they must be allowed to express that fury, and if they are terrified they must be comforted by the staff of the residential home, as well as by the family.

Most social services departments have a process of initial review of the new resident after a fixed period of time. This is linked to payment of fees to the care provider, but it is also a useful opportunity for the social worker to talk about the move with all parties concerned. This process may have to be extended until a point is reached where the person with dementia accepts that this is where they now live.

The social worker needs to remember, in order to be able to help the family, that it is a fact that most people do settle eventually in a residential or nursing care home. Human beings are surprisingly resilient and adaptable, and people with dementia are no different to anyone else in this respect. Their adjustment may be aided by the family making a life history book to bring with them into the long-term care home (Haight

1998, p.85), or creating a collage of significant people, places and events in their life to hang on the wall in their bedroom.

### Helping the carer to adjust to the change

Social workers should remember that the point where someone does come to accept that the residential care home is where they now live is often extremely painful for carers, particularly for their partner. However, they may be reluctant to admit it because it might look as if they do not appreciate the care which is offered by the home. Again, people have to handle a complicated mixture of emotions at this time.

## The death of the person with dementia

Finally we come to the point where the person with dementia dies. At this point the statutory health and social care system has to let go. Resources do not allow for ongoing support to be provided for the carer – and it is difficult to imagine that public funding could ever be available for this service.

A person who has cared for someone close to them with dementia will have lived through a uniquely long-drawn-out process of bereavement. This may have lasted for as long as twenty years in the case of Alzheimer's disease. If people do survive that long they are likely to have reached the final stages of physical and mental deterioration. The social worker should be aware that the partner may have said 'goodbye' to the person many years before. The son or daughter may feel that their mother or father actually left them some time ago. The process known as 'anticipatory grieving' is of particular relevance in this context. Bere Miesen (1997) talks about 'a frustrating contra-diction, a dramatic antithesis. Relatives have to say goodbye slowly to a beloved person who is still there' (p.74). He goes on to say that 'professional care-givers must be trained to deduce from the family's overt behaviour what stage of grieving they are in' (p.77).

Some carers seem to make the long-term care home into a second home, and visit their relative very frequently indeed. This may be a coping strategy which they have developed over the long period of the changing relationship, or it may be a simple desire to continue the relationship, even though the person no longer lives with them. If we are to embrace the idea of a partnership in long-term care between the family and the provider, then it will be understood by the staff of the home that the death of the person also means a further interruption of the daily rhythms of the carer's life.

Unfortunately, care management does not allow social workers time and resources to work with carers before the death, and certainly does not afterwards. This task is probably best undertaken by the carers' support networks of an organization such as the Alzheimer's Society, or one of the generic voluntary organizations that work with carers, such as The National Association of Carers, or Carers National. CRUSE – a voluntary organization that offers bereavement counselling – is another useful resource. Many towns have local carers' projects. There is a considerable body of experience in this field. In addition to the national Alzheimer's Society carers' helpline, there are many local helplines run by local branches. There is now also a national helpline for same-sex carers, which can be reached through the Alzheimer's Society.

## SUMMARY

- For a statutory health and social care support system to work properly for people with dementia and their carers, the support has to be available throughout the whole course of the journey.

- The journey through dementia is different for each person. The journey may last for several years. There are various points on the journey where it may join the pathway of social services care provision.

- We know that the point of diagnosis, the first acceptance of services from outside the family, the contact with respite services within the community, long-term care and the eventual death of the person are places where this meeting of pathways may take place.

- Ease of access, and the speed and sensitivity of the response to the request for help at these points of special need, is crucial to the quality of the social-work service being offered.

- People with dementia and those who care for them have specialized needs. In order to be effective, social workers need additional training to equip them for the task.

# CHAPTER THREE

# The Historical and Legal Context

## INTRODUCTION

The purpose of this chapter is to examine the process by which the role of social work has been developed and redeveloped as new political ideas have evolved. It attempts to answer the question 'How did we get to the place where we are today?'

The main pieces of legislation which prescribe the role for social work in relation to people with dementia are outlined in brief, as a means of helping social workers to understand the basis of their roles and tasks. Most of these laws relate to the duty of care which local authorities hold towards vulnerable adults and/or older people.

The existence of these laws presents social workers with an ongoing challenge to carry out all the tasks which they are given by their local authority, and to maintain a high standard of social work practice. The tensions and challenges posed by this issue are discussed in the latter part of this chapter.

## A BRIEF HISTORICAL OVERVIEW OF SOCIAL WORK WITH OLDER PEOPLE IN THE UK

The provision of personal social services by statutory and voluntary organizations is a feature of all complex industrial societies. The tasks carried out by social workers have been broadly similar in all these societies because they have developed from an attempt by the state to meet the same universal human needs. It was judged that these were the needs which could not be met within the family, by informal community support or by charitable endeavour. The provision of social work amounts to recognition of the collective responsibility which a society accepts for its vulnerable members. The scope and extent of the services provided clearly depends on the society and historical context in which social workers function.

> The social services function derives from the original role of the parish council that was responsible for the administration of the Poor Law, (passed in the reign of Queen Elizabeth 1). That law was the beginning of the concept of the basic safety net that would, when a person was at the end of the line, keep them from falling into the gutter. (Brayne and Martin 1990, p.16)

## The creation of the welfare state

In the United Kingdom the period after the Second World War saw the development of the welfare state. At that time and for the next forty years there was a national consensus that

> The state has an obligation to provide comprehensive services to respond to the problems of poverty, old age and disability, whatever their cause. All citizens have a right to these services – and should not be left to depend on informal, voluntary or private provision, which might operate unevenly and inequitably. (Barclay Report 1982, p.103)

In 1948 the National Assistance Act and the Children Act was passed and laid the foundation upon which future social work was built. It created departments to meet the needs of the different client groups: the children's department, the welfare department and the health department.

There has been a dominant argument since that time that social work should not be involved in any significant way in the giving of financial relief to its clients, even though many of them are living in poverty. That role is taken by the social security system. The crucial requirement for skilled assessment and counselling, however, was to be met by social workers.

This system of different, specialized departments (such as the large child welfare departments) serving the needs of children and adults with particular needs was not without its problems:

> There were difficulties about the distribution of resources; the departmental divisions led to over-narrow assessment of problems and definition of responses. Different officials operating incompatible policies might visit the same family, ignorant of the involvement and plans of others. Individual people were not seen sufficiently as part of their family and social context. (Barclay Report 1982, p.105)

## The Seebohm Report

Twenty years later, social work was reviewed again by central government. Lord Seebohm's review and his subsequent report led to the Local Authority Social Services Act 1970. A legal duty was then imposed on each local authority to provide a generic social services department operating from area offices. These large social services departments immediately attracted more resources, and more social workers were recruited and trained (Barclay Report 1982, p.107).

Many of those recruited were long-established hospital social workers (the descendants of the 'lady almoners' of former times). This remained an area where there was a marked difference in structure between social services departments, which responded to the Seebohm Report in different ways. Generic training of social workers replaced the specialist training undertaken before Seebohm. It was a time of expansion for social work.

Local authorities were also charged to discover 'unmet need' in the geographical area for which they responsible. Public expectation also rose with the creation of the social services area offices, and legislation laid new duties on local authorities. Although roles and tasks were redefined, the tools used by social workers to complete those tasks remained much the same as they had been since the profession first developed.

There was an emphasis, both in training and practice, on the development of counselling skills, mostly following the person-centred, nonjudgmental approach developed by the psychotherapist Carl Rogers, described as:

> probably the most important humanist writer on therapy to have an influence on social work. His impact is, however, indirect, since his greatest significance is in the related field of counselling work and training that has moved his ideas into social work. (Payne 1991 p.169)

## The Barclay Report

The Secretary of State for Social Services approached the National Institute for Social Work in 1980 to conduct another independent review of the roles and tasks of social workers. This led to the publication of the Barclay Report in 1982. In the introduction to the Report the following statement is made, clearly pointing to the fact that some of today's problems have been with us for a long time:

> Social work is a relatively young profession. It has grown rapidly as the flow of legislation has greatly increased the range and complexity of its work ... [social workers] operate uneasily on the frontier between what appears to be almost limitless needs on the one hand and an inadequate pool of resources to meet those needs on the other. (Barclay Report 1982, p.7)

Among other things the report stated that

We believe it is essential that social workers continue to be able to provide counselling and we use the word to cover a range of activities in which an attempt is made to understand the meaning of some event or state of being to an individual, family or group and to plan, with the person or people concerned, how to manage the emotional and practical realities which face them. Such work is always part of assessment and may be a large or small part of future meetings between client and social worker. (p.41)

Counselling was regarded by social workers themselves as the hallmark of their calling (p.41). The relationship between social worker and client was seen as comparable to that between therapist/counsellor and client, and was to be safeguarded by confidentiality in a similar way. (This model of one social worker and one client is one of the few elements of the social work role which has not been revisited and still persists to the present day in adult services.)

The social worker would expect to work with people on an individual basis or within families to facilitate 'movement' in the same way as therapists and counsellors. In the Barclay Report social work was described as short- or long-term:

About 8% of those who come to social services departments become long-term clients. The actual length of time they remain in contact with the department varies greatly from several months to a number of years. They fall into two major groups. Those suffering from chronic physical or mental conditions, and families where children are 'at risk'. (p.15)

Another quote from the Barclay Report states, 'Direct social work tasks include assessment, giving practical services and advice, surveillance and taking control, acting as intermediary and counselling' (p.12).

During the 1970s and 1980s different governments attempted to define the duty of care towards vulnerable citizens

– both children and adults – placed upon local authorities through social services departments.

## The Griffiths Report

Central government commissioned another review of the work of social services only six years after the Barclay Report. It was driven to a large extent by concern about the massive amount of public money which was being spent on social services.

> The 1980s ended with a higher proportion of old people in residential care than at the beginning of the decade, in spite of explicit policies of supporting them in their own home. (Utting 1997, p.284)

The Griffiths report was published in 1988, setting out the framework for the development of the new policy of community care:

> It sought to harness the resources of the health and social services, along with those of the private and voluntary sectors, behind the concept of family-based care, wherever possible in people's own homes. In making a clear distinction between health and social care and confirming that health care alone should fall within the free-at-the-point-of-use NHS, it also raised the spectre of people having to pay for their care if they looked outside their immediate family and neighbourhood networks. (Dalley 1996, p.6)

Griffiths reported back to central government with the recommendation, widely believed at the time to be unpopular with government, that local authorities were the only bodies with the experience and infrastructure to implement the new, reforming policy of Community Care. The report led to the passing of the NHS and Community Care Act 1990. The social services part of the legislation was not enacted until 1993. This is discussed in the next part of this chapter.

It can be seen that social work has been in a long period of transition as governments of different political persuasions attempt to meet challenges, some of which are new and some of which have been an intrinsic part of social work since it first began. A solution to the challenge of finding an affordable way to support old people who need care in order to maintain their independence in their own homes, instead of moving them into long-term care, continues to prove elusive, in spite of strenuous attempts by different governments to implement community care policies.

The social worker working today within the field of dementia, does so within a legislative framework which exists to protect and care for vulnerable adults, as distinct from children.

## SOCIAL CARE LEGISLATION

In addition to the main pieces of legislation (discussed in the following pages) determining the social worker's duty of care towards vulnerable adults, various Acts were passed between 1968 and 1986. These are:

1.  The Health Services and Public Health Act 1968

2.  The Local Authority Social Services Act 1970

3.  The National Health Service Act 1977

4.  The Health and Social Services and Social Security Adjudications Act 1983

5.  The Registered Homes Act 1984

6.  The Disabled Persons (Services, Consultation and Representation) Act 1986. (Brayne and Martin 1992, p.200)

The four key pieces of legislation determining the roles and tasks of social workers working with people with dementia are:

1.  The National Assistance Act 1948

2.      The Chronically Sick and Disabled Persons Act
        1977

3.      The Mental Health Act 1983

4.      The National Health Service and Community
        Care Act 1990

It is important to be clear that, before taking any action in relation to a client, social workers must ask whether they have the legal power to intervene in a particular way, rather than merely a moral obligation. This is a distinction which is often misunderstood by other health care professionals who may have unrealistic expectations of the power of the social worker in a given situation.

## The National Assistance Act 1948

As we have seen, this was the law which was the cornerstone for the creation of the social care part of the welfare state. It places a duty on all local authorities to care for vulnerable members of society, including the elderly. Section 21 of Part 3 of the Act allows the local authority to provide 'residential accommodation for persons who by reason of age, infirmity or any other circumstances are in need of care and attention, which is not otherwise available to them'. (Local authority residential care used to be known by social workers as 'Part 3 accommodation'). A standard charging rate for local authority residential homes is set under Section 22 of the Act. Section 29 of the Act defined vulnerable people as those who are 'substantially or permanently handicapped by illness, injury or congenital deformity'. Local authorities became major providers of services for these vulnerable groups of people and this provider role lasted for the next thirty-five years.

Section 47 of the National Assistance Act relates to compulsory removal from home. In order to apply it, certain conditions have to be met:

(a) the person has to be suffering grave chronic disease or, being aged, infirm or physically incapacitated, is living in insanitary conditions and

(b) is unable to devote to themselves, and is not receiving from other persons, proper care and attention.

The community physician must supply to the court a certificate that he or she has made enquiries and considers that it is necessary to remove the person from the premises where they are, either because:

(a) it is in the interest of that person; or

(b) removal will prevent injury to someone else's health, or prevent a serious nuisance being caused to someone else.

This is a draconian procedure. (There is no legal aid for the person who is to be removed, there is not even any requirement for the person to be represented or even to have legal advice.) For these reasons Section 47 of the National Assistance Act is rarely used now.

Social workers in the field of dementia care need to be aware of it, however, as other professionals may advocate that it should be used in a crisis for a person with dementia. It was under the National Assistance Act that the local authority was given responsibility for ensuring the safety of the property and possessions of a person who is away from home because of an admission to residential or hospital care. Social workers who work with older people will be familiar with carrying out a 'protection of property' procedure under these circumstances.

## The Chronically Sick and Disabled Persons Act 1977

As we have seen, Section 29 of the National Assistance Act lists all people who are deemed to be vulnerable, including age as a criterion of vulnerability. In this piece of legislation local authorities were required to research the population of vulnerable adults in their area and keep a register of them. They were required to assess the needs of this group. Practical help, which was offered under the Act, usually consisted of the provision of meals, assistance in the home, assistance with telephones and equipment necessary to use them, some help with holidays (very rare these days), assistance with travel arrangements for the purpose of obtaining the services which are provided, and works of adaptation to a person's home. The Act also provided for the issue of the orange car-parking badges for disabled drivers/passengers.

Section 29 clients, the mentally disordered and physically ill and the elderly, had to be offered home help and laundry facilities if they were assessed as being needed. Although the local authorities were told that these services were mandatory, they were left with a wide discretion about how this should be done. The law was clearly framed for people with a physical disability. An example of this is the fact that carers of people with dementia sometimes found it difficult to obtain the orange parking badges or access to the 'Dial-A-Ride' schemes which developed in the 1990s.

Assistance with payment of TV licences was introduced. This became more honoured in the breach than the observance but is now being restored by central government.

Social workers who are still working within the framework of the Chronically Sick and Disabled Persons Act 1977 may have to act as advocates/interpreters for their clients in this respect. People with dementia living on their own are unlikely to be able to claim the assistance to which they are entitled. This is a good example of how the special needs of adults who are mentally rather than physically impaired were not considered when these laws were framed. Being framed for people with physical disabilities, the law has not always been easy to apply to people with dementia.

## The Mental Health Act 1983

It is important for all social workers who work with people with dementia to have a basic understanding of the Mental Health Act, even if they do not act as Approved Social Workers. It is only possible here to touch briefly on a few important sections of the Act which are of particular relevance to the field.

This Act is the only means offered within the legal framework of England and Wales, as it presently exists, for the protection of persons whose mental capacity is impaired through dementia. The difficulty in applying the Act to people with dementia has been known for many years and the reforms proposed by the government are very welcome.

In order for the Mental Health Act to apply, the person concerned has to be 'suffering from mental disorder of a nature or degree which warrants the detention of the patient in a hospital for assessment (or for assessment followed by medical treatment) for at least a limited period'. In addition 'he ought to be so detained in the interests of his own health or safety or with a view to the protection of other persons' (Brayne and Martin 1990, p.218).

### Section Two (for assessment) should initially be used in preference to any other Section

The Codes of Practice which have been issued in recent years stress that it is always good practice for people who have to be detained under the Act, to be detained – at least initially – under Section Two of the Act for the purpose of assessment. People cannot be detained under Section Two for longer than 28 days.

### The care programme approach

The care programme approach, which was implicit in Section 117 of the Act, only began to be implemented effectively from the early 1990s. This fresh impetus followed several high-profile cases in which people suffering from mental illness injured or killed other people or themselves and raised public anxiety about care in the community. The intention is to ensure that professionals from different departments work together for the good of the patient. As a result of its implementation social workers are more aware that people detained under Sections 2 and 3 (the Treatment Order, which lasts for six months) have a legal right to regular care and review. Under Section 117 of the Act a key worker must be appointed (GP, social worker or community psychiatric nurse) who may not discharge the case until a proper care package of appropriate services has been set up for the client. The process has to be monitored and reviewed and the case cannot be closed until a care programme approach case conference has been held.

## Guardianship

Guardianship (Section 7 of the Act), which would appear to be the section most suitable for use with adults who lack mental capacity, has proved to be of limited use because of the lack of a 'power to convey' and also the fact that, as in Section 3, the nearest relative has to agree with its use.

It is clear that those who drafted the Mental Health Act of 1983 did not have dementia in mind. The focus was on what we have learned to call 'functional mental illness' and on learning disability.

The Act sometimes has to be used, in spite of its short-comings, if a person with dementia poses such a danger to themselves and/or other people that they can no longer be maintained in the community. It does at least have the merit that the professionals concerned – the consultant psychiatrist, the GP and the Approved Social Worker – have to record the reasons for their decision. They also have to tell the person honestly that they lack the capacity at present to make an informed judgement about the viability of maintaining their life situation as it is at present.

The alternative to using the Mental Health Act is to move people with dementia from their own homes (if they can no longer be supported in the community) without telling them where they are going or why. People are still being taken to residential homes under the impression that they are to stay for a short time and will soon be returning home. Apart from being ethically questionable, this causes confusion and distress to the person and also makes life very difficult for staff at the residential home who have to care for them. Sometimes it is best to use the Mental Health Act if the behaviour of the person with dementia proves to be unmanageable in the community – in cases, for example, where the dementia coexists with functional mental illness.

## The National Health Service and Community Care Act 1990

The NHS and Community Care Act was passed after the Griffiths Report had investigated the current state of social care in considerable detail. It was intended to redress the perceived power imbalance between professional purchasers and providers of care and 'consumers' of care, and to return decision-making to the people who were receiving help. Therefore, people were no longer to be referred to as 'clients' but were to be called 'customers' or 'service users'. The social-work task was redefined in a radical way in 1993 when the social services part of the NHS and Community Care Act 1990 was enacted.

The new roles and responsibilities of social workers have been consolidated into the creation of a system of 'care management' in which the central tasks are:

1. Assessment of the circumstances of the user, including any support required by carers

2.    Negotiation of a care package in agreement with users, carers and relevant agencies, designed to meet identified need with available resources

3.    Implementation and monitoring of the agreed package together with a review of outcomes and any necessary revision of services provided. Social Services Inspectorate 1990 cited in Connolly 1997, p.297)

This is a far cry from the description of the roles and tasks of the social worker in the Barclay Report, published a mere eight years earlier.

Four years later it was possible to see more clearly what was happening in the field.

Care in the community or 'community care' has come to represent both a philosophy and a policy in the United Kingdom with respect to the provision of personal social services for adults. It is important to distinguish between the two. (Seed and Kaye 1994, p.5)

These authors describe four elements which were included in the philosophy of community care:

(a) Quality of life – including material, social and spiritual well-being in a safe environment.

(b) Individualisation, an integrated and individualised response to assessed needs.

(c) Participation – meaning a participatory approach to the provision of services which emphasised personal choice and developing potential.

(d) Developing potential – which meant that support should be built on existing or potential support networks of family, friends and community. (p.5)

Social policy in the 1980s also had a profound effect on the decision to implement the policy of 'care in the community'. The following elements are identified by Seed and Kaye:

1. The closing down of some long-stay hospitals, and reduction in size of others.

2. A redefinition of the role of local authority services from main provider of facilities to enabler or facilitator.

3. Assessments being framed in terms of client needs instead of the parameters of the services available from a given source.

4. The quest for 'value for money' in the provision of appropriate services pursued by various means including:

    (a) Separation between service purchasers and providers

    (b) Monitoring and inspection of services. (p.6)

These factors working in combination had a profound effect on the profession, and the social-work task was redefined in a fundamental way. Now that some years have elapsed since the Act was passed, it is easier to see the intractable nature and complexity of many of the problems, which it attempted to address. Alison Petch cites five key points which illustrate this fact:

1. Community care is not only or even primarily about closing institutions; the majority of community care users have always lived 'outwith' the hospital.

2. Community care is not necessarily cheaper than the institutional alternative. All cost information must be treated with care to ensure comparability.

3.      The needs of community care groups span the health/social care boundary; it is often difficult and inappropriate to separate out the various components.

4.      Multidisciplinary working, including collaboration with GPs, is the key to the effective implementation of community care.

5.      Users and carers should be regarded as active partners in care. (Petch 1997, p.327)

## THE SEMINAR ON COMMUNITY CARE HELD BY THE ROYAL COMMISSION FOR LONG-TERM CARE

The Royal Commission reported back to central government in 1999. As well as publishing a report entitled *With Respect to Old Age* (Sutherland 1999), the Royal Commission also held a seminar to establish the extent to which the community care reforms of 1993 had achieved their objectives. This is a recent, independent assessment of the effect which the reforms have had in practice. It is often hard to see the results of legislation until some time has passed; and this evaluation is of interest to social workers in the field of dementia care, who may derive comfort from the fact that many of the frustrations of their working lives have been validated by the findings of the Royal Commission. It is interesting to remind ourselves how long some of these problems have been in existence.

The following six points are a summary of the Royal Commission's findings.

1.      There has been more home care provided but it is targeted at the most dependent. It was felt that prevention had been squeezed out.

2.      Carers had been helped little, and often services were not being offered in cases where a carer was in evidence.

3.      An over-supply in the residential sector and the effect of local authority purchasing power meant that costs were low, and this made residential care seem attractive in cost terms compared to home care. In effect, it is cheaper to keep a person in long-term residential care than to keep them at home, where they usually wish to remain.

4.      There was also concern about quality in the residential sector overall.

5.      There had been some changes in management culture in social services, but there is still a long way to go to ensure more of a client-based, rather than a service-based, approach.

6.      The division of responsibility between NHS and social services – the health/social divide – caused a number of problems in terms of responsibility and accountability, and perverse cost incentives to take a short-term view based on cost alone remained.

It is encouraging to note that legislation which recognizes the needs of carers and requires social services departments to meet those needs has recently been passed, although it has been a long time coming.

There are two recent Acts of which social workers need to be aware:

## The Carers (Recognition and Services) Act 1995

This Act gave carers statutory recognition and the right to a separate assessment of need if they requested it. It failed, however, to give them the right to provision of support services.

Its impact on carers' access to services seems to have been patchy.

## The Carers Act 2000

The full title of this Act is the Carers and Disabled Children's Act. It gives local authorities power to provide services directly to carers. It also gives them the power to give vouchers to the carer or user for short breaks. It empowers local authorities to provide direct payments to carers in lieu of services. It also enables them to charge carers for services which they receive. (The wording of this clause is unclear, and the voluntary organizations which represent carers are concerned because it is not clear whether local authorities will still be able to charge for respite care (Alzheimer's Society – Public Affairs Section 2000).) The government has provided some new money for carers as part of its modernization of social services initiative.

It is very obvious that there are fewer laws to protect vulnerable adults than there are to protect children. This may partly be because successive governments have been confused about the extent to which the state should intervene in the life of adults. But it must also reflect the ageism which is endemic in our society.

The new factor for our client group is that there is now political recognition that we live in a country with a rapidly ageing population. 'Grey power' means that governments are starting to realize that older people are also voters. So governments have to take the needs of this group more seriously than they have ever done before. At the same time it is hoped that, just as carers emerged as a distinct group during the 1980s, younger people with dementia will also be identified as a subgroup whose own specific needs have to be addressed. There is a real issue about where they should be placed as a client group in order to ensure that they receive the best service.

There is a legal dimension to the social work role with all client groups. With some client groups, e.g. in child protection and mental health, this has always been very clear. This aspect of the role has been less clear for social workers who work in teams for older people because, as we have seen, there are so few statutory duties to protect vulnerable adults.

## OLD TENSIONS AND NEW CHALLENGES FACING SOCIAL WORKERS
### The tension between care and control

The fact that these laws exist, imperfect though they may be, underlines a dilemma which all social workers face at some stage of their career. It has been part of social work since it first became a function of government. Most social workers enter this field – one of the so-called 'caring professions' – from a desire to help and support the less fortunate members of society. However, social workers in social services departments are essentially government employees. In certain roles – notably child protection and mental health – social workers are acting as 'soft policemen'. The element of 'surveillance and control' was included in the description of the roles and tasks of social workers outlined in the Barclay Report (1982, p.12).

> There would probably be wide agreement that social work has a social control function, in that one of its tasks is to promote conformity with what Pearson (1975, p.129) calls '... the binding obligations of civil society'. (Payne 1991, p.204, quoting Pearson 1975)

Each social worker has to sort out the conflicting demands of the caring role and the law-enforcement role for him/herself. The tensions which have always existed within the profession between, on the one hand, the drive towards compassion and care for the weak and disadvantaged members of society, and, on the other hand, its assessment, rationing and enforcement role are still with us.

In spite of the seismic shift which has taken place, traditional social work values still survive.

As commercial and contractual relations penetrate social work agencies themselves, as practitioners are required to assess service users for individualised packages of care, treatment, training, containment or punishment and as their work comes under ever more detailed state regulation and surveillance, social work still strives and yearns for the caring, intimate, inclusive, voluntary, negotiated, co-operative, trusting and empowering relationships on which its golden years of expansionism were built. This is not an irrational, backward-looking fantasy; as an organised activity, social work only makes sense if it can be done within just such an ethos, and is only efficient and equitable on these terms. (Jordan 1997, p.10)

## The tension between the need to preserve confidentiality and the duty to protect the vulnerable

Confidentiality is another issue which has always been of great significance to social workers, and confusion about the tension discussed in the previous section led to lack of clarity of roles. Several high-profile child abuse cases in the 1980s, and the 'scapegoating' of social workers by the media which followed, did achieve more clarification of this area of social work practice. In 1987 the Access to Personal Files Act was passed, which meant that clients could (under certain circumstances) read what social workers had written about them. This coincided with the introduction of computerization into social services departments, which meant that social work recording fell within the remit of the Data Protection Act. This gradually led to a very different style of recording than the 'process recording' which social workers had used until then. The important issue of confidentiality had always been a difficult area for social work. The simple proposition that the source of a social worker's information is confidential has always been accepted. Without it, people would not be prepared to give information to social workers to protect the vulnerable. However, there are certain cases, such as where the social worker is told that a child is being abused, where confidentiality cannot be assured.

Until the mid-1990s the emphasis was all on the protection of children. Nowadays social workers are much more aware of the need to protect vulnerable adults as well. Now, for example, all social services departments have elder abuse policies and procedures. Social workers are now much more aware that some adults are as vulnerable as children, and people with dementia are certainly included in their number.

## The debate about generic or specialist training for social workers

Before 1970, when the recommendations of the Seebohm Report were implemented, social workers were trained to work in the specialist fields mentioned above. Post-Seebohm the Central Council for Education and Training in Social Work became responsible for generic training of social workers, so that all social workers, in whatever field they practiced, received the same training, and skills were held to be transferable. Experience with a particular client group was gained on the job, and social workers became familiar only with the specific pieces of legislation which affected their clients.

There was a strong commitment to generic training within the profession. As in the debates about care versus control, and confidentiality, the debate about generic versus specialist training was strongly informed by the issue of child protection. It became apparent that social workers could have been described as 'Jacks and Jills of all trades and masters of none' and that some areas, notably child protection and mental health social work, required further specialist training.

So far no specialist training has been universally provided for working with clients with dementia. Work in this field was historically seen as bolted-on to care of the elderly, even though the increasing number of people with dementia who were being referred to teams for older people was known. A study (Moriarty and Webb 1997) of three social services departments found that the area teams (not specialist community mental health teams) were receiving three to five referrals per month concerning older people with dementia.

Another problem was that there was always uncertainty as to whether dementia should be placed in services for older people or in mental health services, and people with dementia received an inadequate service because of this. In many instances they fell between the two groups and through the social care net altogether. Social-work training adopted a competence-based model from the mid 1980s onwards: 'Competence is a wide concept which embodies the ability to transfer skills and knowledge to new situations within the occupational area' (The Training Agency 1988, quoted in Evans 1997, p.356). This is the same approach as is used in the National Vocational Qualification (NVQ), and emphasis is placed on the ability of the social-work student to demonstrate competence in different areas of practice.

In the mid-1990s the inadequacy of completely generic training for social workers was acknowledged and the 'preferred pathway' route was introduced into the new Diploma in Social Work (DipSW) which replaced both the old Certificate of Qualification in Social Work (CQSW) and the less academic Certificate in Social Services (CSS). This latest approach requires students to identify the client group with which they hope to work during their training. There is not yet a nationally accepted module specific to dementia within the DipSW course, although there are various post-qualification courses available at university level and through some dementia services development centres.

Bradford Dementia Group has pioneered the Certificate in Dementia Care.

## The change from welfare to the social market

A new challenge for social workers has been the change from the welfare model, where almost all social care was provided by local authorities, to the market model of care. Until the late 1990s the paradigm of 'the market' was embraced, with varying degrees of enthusiasm, within the NHS and Social Services. The difficulty of applying this doctrine to human beings began to be experienced very soon after the NHS and Community Care Act was passed. Social workers, working at the coalface, knew that it was not possible to make a legitimate comparison between purchasing services to meet the needs of human beings, in all their diversity and frailty, and purchasing goods in a supermarket, which seemed to be the preferred model of the government of the day. Recognition of the inadequacy of the social care system has been made with the provision, during 1999–2000, of new monies from central to local government under the prevention grants and careers grants.

The idea that bad providers of social care would be forced out of the market by competition has been found to be an oversimplification. The purchasers of services (whether they are social services departments acting on behalf of their customers, or private individuals) do not have a range of products from which to choose. Certainly the gulf between the NHS and social services sometimes seems as wide as ever, and the two cultures are still deeply entrenched behind their own barricades. The process of integration still has a long way to go, but the idea that 'the market' somehow exerts a benign influence of its own accord on the population has failed to convince the electorate.

If a person with dementia needs a long-term care place, they usually need it urgently and they go where there is a vacancy. There is no guarantee that the vacancy is in a place which can offer them the best care for their needs at that time. The lack of social services resources means that those who are eligible for public funding and cannot purchase care without it may have to wait for funding. This means that when the money is available, people are not likely to turn down the offer of a place, even if the residential home may not be able to offer the best quality care. People who can afford to pay for their own care can do so as soon as it is needed – so there is, as there always was, one rule for those who can pay and another for those who cannot.

The model for the division between purchasers and providers within the health and social care system has continued to evolve.

After the change of administration in 1997 the government proposed a shift in emphasis in the NHS and social services towards a model of 'integrated care'. In other words, there was recognition that the divisions created by the internal market caused their own problems. The phrase 'joined-up government' has become popular. From 1997 onwards the creation of primary care groups (later trusts), made up of clusters of GPs and others in a locality, replaced fundholding GPs as purchasers.

The effects of changes which started in the 1990s will take several years to become apparent. It seems unlikely, however, that there will be a return to the social work world as it was before 1993. There is clearly no intention to revert to the former situation where local authorities, between 1948 and 1993, were major providers of 'in-house' social care services. The days of large numbers of residential homes, home care services and day centres run by the social services departments have apparently gone forever. Those services have proved too expensive to maintain.

There were pockets of good practice within some social services departments which had built up considerable expertise over the years in looking after people with special needs such as dementia. That expertise has now been either lost or dispersed, which is a sad and unforeseen result of the change in social policy.

The market-place has been introduced into the provision of care for vulnerable people and seems to be here to stay. In this respect it may be said that the population at large has accepted the reforms of the Conservative administration of the 1980s and 1990s. No political party appears to have plans to return to the situation as it was before 1993.

> 'Market welfare' has partly replaced 'state welfare'. But we still have care in the community as an expression of social policy in recognition of what we may call a continuing (and in some respects even a growing) sense of shared social responsibility. The tension between hard-nosed economics or finance, and altruism, is very great. This is the context for understanding what care in the community means and how social workers, health care staff and others perceive, and try to carry out, new tasks. (Seed and Kaye 1994, p.6)

This analysis, which was made in 1994, remains true six years later, even though the government today is of the opposite ideological persuasion from the one that passed the NHS and Community Care Act.

The demographic fact of an ageing population which makes increasing demands on the social and health care system, combined with ever-rising public expectations, is forcing the United Kingdom to re-examine the system which was developed in 1948.

> Demographic patterns suggest much larger numbers of people living alone in old age. Smaller families, marriage breakdown, differences in life expectancy between men and women, geographical variations in the distribution of older people will affect the kind of health and social care services we will need. (Cayton 1997, p.54)

The country simply cannot afford to provide 'cradle to grave' social and health care from the public sector without raising taxation to levels which would apparently be unacceptable to the electorate.

The social care market-place now consists of a variety of providers. In the continuing care field, for example, there are some very large, independent, corporate businesses, some medium-sized, and some small, family-run businesses (which appear to be under threat in the present financial climate). Some of the voluntary groups who provide continuing care have emerged as significant providers. There are also various 'not for profit' companies (many of them formed from the former local authority provision in a local area). In some areas there is still a 'rump' of local authority provision.

A decade after the NHS and Community Care Act there is a different financial climate in the independent sector. Recent European legislative changes such as the introduction of the National Minimum Wage and the Working Time Directive have increased the cost of staffing residential and nursing homes. There is now a clear trend towards mergers and takeovers, which has led to the creation of large, corporate companies. The current climate is inhospitable for the small, private providers of residential and nursing care. Social workers have become 'care managers'.

Social workers in the field of dementia care are functioning within this legislative framework, which has grown up in a rather piecemeal fashion since 1948. Their task is now clearly confined, under the community care legislation, to the four core tasks outlined on pages 51–52. They are only allowed to work with clients who meet the eligibility criteria agreed on by their local authority. (The NHS and Community Care Act made the introduction of these criteria mandatory.) Ongoing work with clients, as visualized by the Barclay Report, is no longer en-visaged as part of the social work task. Social workers have been redesignated as care managers in order to clarify this change of role.

Social workers who work with children and families and within child protection still undertake long-term work. So do those who work with adults with certain disabilities. But the system does not allow those who work with older people to do so. The reason given for this is that there are so many older people who need assessment that there would be no time to complete new assessments if long-term work were undertaken. The number of older people in need of social work intervention is far larger than in any other client group, and a high percentage of all work undertaken by social service departments is with older people. However, my experience leads me to believe that this model (of undertaking short-term work only) is failing people with dementia and those who care for them. It does not, and cannot, meet their needs for ongoing support over a period, often, of several years.

## National care standards

The creation of a social market with a 'mixed economy of care' has made the question of registration and inspection of providers of social care extremely important. Previously there was an anomalous situation whereby local authorities registered and inspected all providers of continuing care, including their own. Home care was not registered or inspected at all.

> Since the purpose of health and social care is improved quality of life for individuals and the community, the state has a role in regulating and defining quality. To do so is to promote both private and public good: private good in that the individual's quality of life is enhanced, public good in improved health in the community and reduction in the overall burden of morbidity. (Cayton 1997, p.56)

The new National Care Standards Commission has powers to investigate complaints and replaces the 150 local authority registration and inspection units. It inspects local authority care establishments for children and vulnerable adults, as well as care provided within the independent and voluntary sector. It is planned to be fully operational by spring 2002 and will, for the first time, provide an independent watchdog for standards of long-term care. For the first time also, there will be a system for the inspection of home care. The National Care Standards Commission will provide this in accordance with legislation enacted in spring 2000, following the publication of the White Paper *Modernising Social Services* (Department of Health 2000a).

It is encouraging to see that dementia care mapping, as developed by the Bradford Dementia Group, is advocated in the *Forget Me Not* report for use in long-term care homes. The report states that

> Dementia Care Mapping (DCM) for monitoring the environment experienced by users can make a great deal of difference. Learning to undertake DCM and getting feedback from it can greatly enhance the awareness and understanding of staff and improve the care they provide. Visits from specialists to monitor the quality of care and support staff can be beneficial for both users and staff. (Audit Commission 2000, p.11)

The report concluded that

> people who would otherwise need residential care could live at home if provided with flexible home-based care provided by joint health and social services teams. They found that most people prefer to be supported in their own homes, if they are given the choice. So, authorities and trusts need to respond to this, by considering a shift in the balance towards community-based care. Using resources differently, to provide more home-based services, could help to meet people's needs more effectively. (p.7)

It is to be hoped that local authorities will heed this report. If they do, social workers in the field of dementia care should be involved in the development of innovative schemes and new partnerships.

## SUMMARY

- In the UK the roles and tasks of social workers are rooted in legislation passed by central government, and their role is closely controlled within the policies of the local authority. Social work has been under sustained review and reorganization since the 1970s as different administrations have tried to tackle the spiralling cost and the shortcomings of welfare provision.

- The key pieces of legislation which affect services to older people are

    The National Assistance Act 1948

    The Chronically Sick and Disabled Persons Act 1977

    The Mental Health Act 1983

    The NHS and Community Care Act 1990

- Other pieces of legislation have been enacted since 1948, affecting the way services are delivered to older people. However, they are very few compared to legislation about protection of and services to children.

- Social workers have faced certain challenges and professional tensions since the creation of the welfare state. The tension between care and control, between the need to preserve confidentiality and the duty to protect the vulnerable, and the debate abut generic versus specialist training have been with us for a long time. Newer challenges facing social workers are the transition from 'welfare' to 'social market' and the increasing importance of regulation in the world of social care.

# CHAPTER FOUR

# Good Practice in Social Work with People with Dementia and Their Carers

## INTRODUCTION

This chapter focuses on the core tasks of social work in relation to people with dementia – assessment, including risk assessment, and care planning. It highlights major challenges and proposes some strategies for meeting these challenges.

Many people over the age of seventy-five are likely to have some mental and/or physical disabilities, which develop as part of the ageing process. These have implications for autonomy and dignity and they need to be understood by all social workers who work with older people.

## GENERIC FACTORS WHICH COMMONLY AFFECT THE LIVES OF OLDER PEOPLE

Most people over seventy-five have some degree of physical impairment. At present, in order to be considered as needing help from social services under the eligibility criteria, older people have to be suffering from a considerable degree of physical and/or mental disability. Age itself is not a sufficient reason for social services to offer assistance.

It is no wonder that many people in this age group suffer from depression, presenting in different degrees of severity. Social workers need to remind themselves that reactive depression is particularly prevalent among older people. This has been demonstrated in many studies. One such study is that conducted by Gurland *et al.* (1983) who studied a sample of 396 individuals over the age of 65, randomly drawn from Greater London. They found that

> Up to a third [of their sample] could be regarded as having some experience of depression, but the most important finding was that 12.4% could be classified as suffering from 'pervasive depression' (depression which pervades most aspects of life and warrants the attention of a mental health professional). (Brayne and Ames 1988, P.19)

Many older people feel the loss of control over their own life very keenly. This is such a frightening issue for most of us that we refuse to contemplate it – linked as it is to the fear of disease and death, the great taboo of our times. We live in a society which pretends that we are all going to remain young, healthy and, preferably, beautiful for the whole of our lives. We are in collective denial about the inevitable loss of physical health and autonomy, which is associated with growing old.

Therefore, no plans are made – no thought is given to what a person would like to happen to them, should they become dependent on other people for their survival. When disability strikes, either suddenly with a stroke or heart attack, or insidiously with chronic illness, the person has to come to terms with the overwhelming fears that may be engendered by losing control of one's own life.

One of the most dominant principles to consider in social work practice is the person's right to be treated with dignity and respect. Their independence must be respected and they have a right to make their own life choices. Generic social work with older people places great emphasis on this.

Unfortunately, many older people suffer from two major misconceptions. In the first place, they think that social workers really want to remove them from their own homes and are empowered to remove them, without their consent, to long-term care homes. The general public is not aware that, since the community care legislation was introduced in 1993, the thrust of social services policy has theoretically been to maintain people in their own homes for as long as possible. In the second place, they are not aware that public funding is no longer readily available to support large numbers of people in long-term care, and that people nowadays have to be very disabled before they qualify for public funding for long-term care.

The model of social work with older people was developed to meet the needs of physically frail older people who are in full possession of their mental faculties. The care management forms are easy to complete with them. The social worker can certainly ask such a person to discuss what they feel they need, whereas this is clearly not always possible with the person with dementia.

## THE ASSESSMENT
### Making contact with the person with dementia

The social worker who works in this field knows that his/her first duty is to gain access to the person's home somehow. This is not always easy when the person is living with a carer, but it is particularly challenging if the person lives alone. The person with dementia cannot be helped unless this is achieved. The social worker has to develop a relationship of trust with him or her.

When a new case is allocated, this is the overriding priority, and the social worker often has to draw on all her/his interpersonal skills and ability and use lateral thinking in order to gain entry to the house and access to the situation. A social worker has no right to go into the home of any adult, whatever their age, if s/he has not been invited.

If a person in possession of their mental faculties refuses to admit the social worker to their home, there is nothing that the social worker can do but leave the premises. If there is reason to believe that an older person is unable to answer the door, e.g. because they have fallen and are lying on the floor, or are ill and in need of care and attention, the social worker has to contact the police. Only the police have the legal right to effect an entry to the property. This applies even if the social worker is an Approved Social Worker acting under the Mental Health Act.

The social worker will also be aware that many people with dementia retain the ability to present a coherent picture of their daily lives which adequately answers the assessment questions. (We used to call this 'confabulation'.) As such they may appear to be managing perfectly well on their own. (A person-centred interpretation of this behaviour would suggest that the person is trying to make sense of the partial information which is being supplied to them by their own damaged brain. They are using coping strategies which formerly worked well to keep prying strangers at bay.) The experienced social worker knows that every effort must be made to preserve the person's self-esteem during the interview, and will avoid intrusive questioning when it becomes clear that the person is unable to answer direct questions. If enough time is taken, the cognitive impairment will be revealed in the course of a conversation. Patience is needed.

The social worker who lacks experience of working in this field is likely to be disconcerted if the person flatly refuses to co-operate. In accordance with 'good practice' for work with older people s/he will go away after the initial visit, write a short report and close the case. S/he may well feel that he has done well to respect the person's independence and right to choose. Unfortunately this still happens far too often.

An alternative and equally common response of the social worker who lacks dementia expertise and experience, and therefore confidence in their own judgement, is that they may be unduly influenced by other people's fear and concern about the person with dementia. S/he may be swept along on a tide of concern for what is considered to be the 'safety' of the person and end up making decisions which are not person-centred and not in their best interest, but which satisfy anxious neighbours.

## Where should assessments be conducted?

There seems to be a consensus in all the professions involved that assessments are best carried out in the person's own home, where they are in familiar surroundings. However, this is not always possible, and some medical assessments are carried out in day hospitals or at hospital outpatient clinics. In these situations the person with dementia may well be disturbed and anxious. Even in their own home they will be aware that they are being judged and found wanting in some way. The situation requires careful handling if it is to yield positive results.

Even if the person is living with a carer the loss of insight caused by the dementia may lead the person to believe that they are managing their own life adequately. They may fight strenuously to prevent what they perceive to be the social worker's unwarranted interference.

## Achieving a balance between respect for autonomy and the imperative to complete the assessment of need

The issue of respect for a person's dignity, privacy and independence has to be balanced by the social worker against the need to convince the person with impaired judgement that they do in fact need help. The person may be hungry because they are forgetting to shop for food, or to eat it if someone else provides it. They may be cold because they have forgotten how to turn on the central heating. They may be vulnerable to abuse of different kinds. But they may still refuse to let the social worker help, unless s/he can manage to win their trust. Never forget that as a social worker you are a complete stranger to the person. You may have to use considerable skill to establish a point of contact upon which to build a relationship of trust.

## How long does the assessment take?

A thorough assessment of the needs of a person with dementia takes time. Social workers will know that the initial assessment visit does not always allow enough time to establish and clarify all the needs of the person with dementia and their carer(s). Even detailed medical assessments can only give us a partial assessment. They are unlikely to be able to tell us easily what the experience of the loss of autonomy caused through cognitive impairment feels like. The person with dementia is likely to find it difficult to define and express their needs to another person. Assessment of a person with dementia, therefore, has to be a dynamic process, evolving over a period of time.

## The need for emotional support to ensure a full assessment

If the assessment of need is to be thorough and accurate, the person with dementia will need considerable emotional support from the social worker as well as carer(s) and/or other providers of care services. People with dementia often find direct questioning something of an ordeal, as they may be unable to provide direct answers. They may expend considerable energy on trying to divert or deflect the person making the assessment in an attempt to conceal the fact that they are unable to answer the question.

Many social workers still struggle with the concept of the need for intervention versus the person's rights to autonomy. We seem to struggle with this issue more than health care professionals, who appear to find it easier to believe in the fact that they are acting in the best interest of the individual, even if the individual makes it very clear that they do not want their help. This is one manifestation of the cultural difference between social services and health care professionals.

Dementia-specific assessment tools are not usually included in the care management documentation used by social services. The Care Needs Assessment Pack (CarenapD) is one tool which has been developed for this purpose (see McWalter 1997, p.157)

The question of how we can meet the challenge of making good assessments of need within the constraints imposed by care management will be discussed further in the next chapter.

## THE CARE PLAN
### Care planning with multiple clients

The traditional social work model derives from the medical model, which works on the principle that you have one social worker who works with one client. This model is still applied to work with older people. Although it is now generally accepted that the needs of carers have to be considered as well, the way that the data is collected from referral forms still indicates the underlying assumption that the client is a single individual – the person with dementia. But the carer may also be the client. If the social worker is allocated a case with a large family whose members are all finding it very hard to accept the diagnosis and even harder to make the necessary decisions, you might have four or five clients.

In family meetings convened to assist the decision-making process, it is commonplace for the person with dementia to disappear metaphorically from the discussion. Old resentments, ongoing sibling rivalry, past family history, can combine in a powerful way. Unless the social worker has the interpersonal skills to deal with a potentially explosive situation, the meeting may deteriorate into mutual recriminations. The conflict will be left unresolved and, more importantly, no decisions will be made.

## Case study 1

Although Mrs Carlton had recently become forgetful and erratic in her behaviour, her married children, Peter, Ann and Richard, were unaware of how cognitively impaired she had become, until Mr Carlton suddenly died from a massive heart attack. All three children felt very guilty when he died, as well as bereaved, because they had not been aware that he was ill and felt they had neglected him. The three children reacted differently to his death and the fact that they now had a very infirm mother to look after.

Peter, who lived nearby, took over the financial management of his mother's life. He consulted his own solicitor and then made an application for her to be placed under the Court of Protection. By doing this he felt that he had discharged his duty to his parents. Richard, who lived a hundred miles away, could not come to terms with his mother's failing mental powers. He managed to avoid any involvement in the situation at all. The hands-on care was left to Ann, the daughter. With a full-time job and three children aged between fourteen and eighteen, she soon began to feel that she could not cope. Her husband David began to resent the time consumed by his mother-in-law's care needs. He became angry with his wife's brothers because they had so little involvement.

Mrs Carlton, bewildered and afraid as a result of her husband's death, became more forgetful and disorientated than ever. She started ringing Ann and Peter many times during the day and night, asking different questions about practical issues and forgetting the answers as soon as they were given.

After two months during which Ann was daily going to see that her mother was all right before work, spending her lunch-break giving her a meal, calling in on the way home as well as answering innumerable phone calls, and doing all the laundry and shopping, the situation broke

## Case study 1 (continued)

down. Ann could no longer carry on. She went to see her doctor because she started crying and was unable to stop. He confirmed that Mrs Carlton had dementia, probably Alzheimer's disease. (Ann learned for the first time that Mr Carlton had been told this diagnosis over a year previously but had chosen not to share this with his children.) The doctor explained that nothing could be done for Mrs Carlton, prescribed Prozac for Ann, and advised her to 'put her mother in a home as soon as possible'.

David immediately called a family conference when he was told this, summoning Richard and his wife Jackie, and Peter and his wife Sue to attend. He was very angry with his wife's brothers, particularly Richard, because they had allowed Ann to carry the burden of caring for their mother virtually on her own. Tempers ran high at this meeting. This was on a Saturday.

The following Monday morning David rang Social Services (eventually obtaining the number from directory enquiries when he was unable to find it in the phone book). He spoke to the switchboard and was told that it was the wrong area office. After two more phone calls he was finally put through to the Elderly Services duty desk. A student social worker picked up the phone, asked David several questions in order to complete the referral form, and said the duty social worker would contact him as soon as she was free. By the time the social worker did make contact, David Carlton was very angry indeed.

Clearly this family will need considerable work and this was not an ideal start. It appears that there are at least two clients here, Mrs Carlton and her daughter Ann. There may be more. The social worker will have to work with the conflicts, which exist within the family if a satisfactory care package is to be created for Mrs Carlton. Crucial decisions will have to be made.

## The need for continuous adjustment to the care plan

The conventional approach to care planning sees it as an exercise which can be completed within a specific time-frame. The model is that, following the initial assessment, the needs of the person are identified and a plan is set out as to how these needs can be met. The assumption is that they can be clearly identified and that, once they have been met through the care plan, the situation will return to stability, allowing the 'case' to be closed.

Experience teaches us, however, that in the case of the person with dementia, situations can change very quickly. There seem to be two reasons for this. One is the progressive nature of the dementia, which means that changes in the person's behaviour continue to occur. The other is that the carer(s) also live in a situation of change. Life for them becomes a long series of little losses, of change after change. The care plan, therefore, needs to be seen as a living, dynamic document. It has to change to meet the needs of the people involved.

The carefully constructed care package frequently has to be altered, with frequent minor changes being made. Families where dementia is present can be like houses of cards. The whole edifice built by the care package can collapse because of something as minor as a case of flu. The social worker in this field has to be able to live and work with the fact that a great deal of hard work completed one week may all have to be done again in a slightly different form in three weeks' time. The whole care plan might have to be completely changed in another month. Flexibility is one of the most important attributes for a social worker who works in this field.

## Case study 2

Mrs Lily Cardington was eighty-three and had lived in the same house for many years. She had no family except a niece who lived fifty miles away. Her behaviour gradually became more and more eccentric. She started to hold long conversations with her dog, about which she told her neighbour. (The dog had died the previous year.) She made meals for her deceased husband and brother each night. Her niece became very concerned about her safety and wanted Lily to move into residential care.

On Christmas Eve Lily left the house at night – in her nightclothes. Her neighbour, Joan, saw her outside when she was going to bed and brought her back. When the same thing happened the next night, Joan became very concerned. The police picked Lily up some distance from her home on two other occasions. The police and the neighbour were convinced that Lily needed to move into residential care. The police contacted the Emergency Duty Team but Lily refused to let the worker in. The same thing happened when the social worker from the specialist team visited, at the request of the police. Lily was extremely suspicious and hostile and shouted abuse through the letterbox.

The social worker then contacted the neighbour, whose phone number was on file, by arrangement. Joan agreed to take the social worker round to visit Lily. By this means the social worker was able to gain admission to the house and to complete an assessment. They had a long talk. It became clear over a cup of tea that Lily was very lonely. The assessment was completed in the form of a friendly chat, with no forms being produced in front of Lily, but being completed by the social worker immediately she returned to the office. The visit lasted over an hour, but the time was well spent in that the initial assessment was completed and Lily agreed to see the social worker again.

## Case study 2 (continued)

The doctor visited at the request of the social worker and found that Lily had a chest infection, which was obviously making her more confused than usual. She responded quickly to antibiotic treatment and when she was feeling better she agreed to allow a home carer to visit her.

A care package was created with home carers calling twice a day and two days spent at the day centre each week. Lily soon became attached to the home carers. Joan – who was also lonely – began to take an interest in Lily and gradually became involved in her care. Later Joan discovered that a neighbour's dog was actually visiting Lily every day while its owners were out at work! The picture of confusion and hallucinations changed, and Lily was revealed as a very lonely woman with mild cognitive impairment, who talked to the dog because she lacked human company. The neighbour and the home carers became her friends, and her well-being was enhanced through a crisis which could, if not properly handled, have led to an inappropriate admission to long-term care. Fortunately Lily's niece, seeing the improvement in her aunt's quality of life, accepted the assessment and co-operated with the care package.

This is an example of a case where the situation was not as it appeared at first, and the assessment was completed over a period of time as events unfolded.

## People are likely to refuse services

The person with dementia who is reluctant
to accept services

The development of the care plan following assessment is a crucial element of the care management task, which is completed as a result of consultation between the client and the social worker. The care plan is available for all interested parties to see and is reviewed at regular intervals. Care planning requires a particular emphasis if the 'client' is a person with dementia who is unable to give informed consent to the plan.

It is extremely common for a person with dementia to refuse services when they are offered, and the social worker should not be disconcerted when this happens. It is important to use the gift of empathy at this point and imagine how the social worker may appear through the eyes of the person with dementia. Because the dementia has caused impaired judgement and insight, the person may honestly believe that they are managing their own life in a satisfactory manner and do not need any outside help. Or, if they do retain some insight, they may see the social worker as someone who is going to interfere, take control and possibly remove them from their own home. The psychological mechanism of 'denial' can be seen operating strongly in people with dementia throughout the relationship with health and social care professionals. It should not be underestimated. Some strategies are here suggested as to how the social worker can persuade the person with dementia to accept services.

Honesty is the best policy as far as possible, but there are occasions when the pace and the way that information is given are extremely important. Information should be given gradually, at the right speed for the person to be able to absorb it.

Find out in advance, from the carer, or another member of the family, or friend, as much as you can about the person. This will enable you to work out which approach – and which person – is likely to elicit the most cooperation from the person with dementia. A home carer who has built up a good relationship with them may be more effective than a social worker in persuading them to accept respite services.

If you are trying to persuade the person with dementia to accept any of the respite services, you might find that the following ideas are helpful:

- Suggest that the carer needs to have a break. Even if s/he does not see the need for respite for himself or herself, the person might be prepared to cooperate for the sake of the carer.

- Suggest that they might like to have a break from their carer. Any couple will 'get on each other's nerves' if they spend all day and every day together, and tensions often arise in these circumstances. Most people are able to agree with this type of approach.

- Suggest that they might like to meet other people of their own age who share their interests. Advocate a change of scene.

- Suggest that 'the doctor' feels they should go. Many people of the oldest generation have a very respectful attitude towards the medical profession and will be much more inclined to 'do what the doctor says' than anybody else – including their family.

- Invite the person to go and have a look at the day care centre or residential home and give their opinion of what it is like.

- Suggest that attending the respite centre might give the person an opportunity to regain their lost confidence in a specialist environment. In my experience, there is no stigma attached to admitting that a person has problems with their memory and they will readily accept that this is so.

- Ask the person to go with the carer for a trial visit to the respite centre.

## The carer who refuses to accept help

The carer of a person with dementia who refuses help is equally hard to work with. This occurs most often with husbands, wives and partners, but does also occur with other people. One reason for the refusal may be that they are in denial, which is as common in carers as it is in people with dementia. It may be that the mechanism of denial is being used because they do not want or are not able to admit to themselves, let alone a stranger, that the problem is so severe that they need help. Admitting this means admitting all sorts of other unpleasant things, such as a problem with accepting that they are no longer in control, a resentment that the professionals are 'taking over', and, of course, guilt. The attachment history of the individuals concerned is likely to be very significant here. (See Chapter Four.)

They may have all sorts of reasons for wanting to keep away those whom they see as representatives of authority. There might be dark reasons, such as an abusive relationship. At the other end of the spectrum it may be that a person who has coped successfully all their lives just cannot face the fact that dementia has defeated them. They may need help to come to terms with the diagnosis, or they may be afraid of a diagnosis being made at all. The following case example illustrates a woman who could not accept either the diagnosis of dementia, or the fact that she needed help from outside the family.

Carers who initially refuse help need careful work, which cannot be hurried. It is skilful work, because if the approach is made without sufficient sensitivity the situation will close – literally as well as metaphorically – with the social worker on one side of the door and the carer on the other. The social worker needs to acknowledge the carer's concern, helping them to talk about their worries and giving them permission to express the negative emotions which they are often experiencing but feel are unacceptable to express to other people

## Case study 3

Mrs. Elsie Broom had looked after her husband, James, at home for two years. He had suffered from kidney failure for some time and was very frail. None of their four children lived locally, but they were a very close family.

When the two daughters visited their parents they became increasingly concerned about their father's mental state. His memory was extremely bad and he was showing distress about this. One daughter tried to talk to her mother, but she would not accept any suggestion that her husband was abnormally confused.

A year later a social worker was asked by the GP to make an assessment. She visited and was able to establish a good rapport with both Elsie and James. Elsie finally admitted that she did know something was wrong. She went to a drawer and produced an unopened envelope from the Alzheimer's Society, dated twelve months previously. Elsie told the social worker that her daughter had contacted the Society for information but that she could not bring herself to open the envelope when it arrived – so she simply put it in a drawer. It had taken a further crisis and the passage of an additional twelve months before she was able to accept help.

Over time she was able to explore her reaction with the social worker. She was able to see that she had always been a woman of great strength and competence who had held her family together through various crises. She could not accept the fact that she was now confronted with something – James' dementia – for which there was no medical treatment. She had to be helped to see that she and her children could learn new skills which they could use to make James' life the best that it could be, and that by learning more about the condition she would feel that she was more in control of the situation.

## The person with dementia who lives alone has special needs which require a special approach

All the strategies suggested in the previous section presuppose that the social worker is able to ascertain which is likely to be the most effective approach, assuming the presence of a carer. The fact is that many people with dementia live alone. However, in my experience, it is relatively rare to find people who have nobody at all who knows and cares about them.

If there is no partner or close family, there are neighbours and friends. Somebody almost always ends up holding the parcel when the music stops. In the absence of family or friends it may be a next-door neighbour with a conscience. Church and community groups are often excellent sources of information and support about individuals who may appear to be totally isolated. Social workers in this field need to develop knowledge about, and contacts with, these informal care networks. It is important to respect the independence of the person with dementia as far as possible, and the person-centred approach to dementia emphasizes the validity of the reality of that person's experience and their rights to behave as they wish. But the social worker needs to find out as much as possible about what the person was like before they developed dementia, in order to help them. This may involve talking to old friends and neighbours as well as family members. If the social worker is creating a care package which involves a stranger coming into the house, or which involves the person with dementia leaving their own home, it is extremely important to find the key to effective communication.

## THE ISSUE OF RISK

The identification and management of risk with all client groups has become a very significant issue for both purchasers and providers of care. This is in response to various cases, in which social workers have been involved, which have attracted considerable public attention. People with dementia are among the most vulnerable adults in our society, particularly if they live alone.

We shall therefore examine some of the issues surrounding risk, in particular the pressure exerted by other professionals and by families to remove a person to long-term care before this is needed, as a means of minimizing risk. Often, the physical security of the person seems to be more important to families than considerations about their well-being.

An assessment of the risks should form part of the social worker's overall assessment. The care plan will demonstrate that these risks have initially been taken into account. It will be amended as the risks change, as they inevitable will as the situation changes.

A discussion of risk must include the issue of abuse.

People who live alone, without any relatives, are particularly vulnerable to the making of wrong decisions by professionals, and their civil rights can easily be eroded. As a group they are the most clearly in need of advocacy. (See p.104.)

When a person with dementia who lives alone is reported to be 'wandering' in the street, there is likely to be an outbreak of anxiety from those who live nearby, as the example of Lily Cardington (case study 2) shows. Social workers have to be very sure of their philosophy, as well as their knowledge base, in order to oppose other professionals as well as relatives and say, 'Steady on – we need to find out more.' Let us ask, for example, the following questions:

- *'What do you mean by wandering?'* 'Wandering' is not a specific term. It may describe several different types of behaviour and implies a lack of purpose, which is insulting.

- *'Has s/he forgotten how to find his/her way home, or has s/he simply forgotten how to open the door?'* If the person has lost their ability to find their way back to their

own home this could place them at risk. If they can
no longer cope with a complicated door lock or
security system this is a practical problem that could
have a practical solution.

- *'Has s/he lost his/her road sense?'* If s/he has not, but is
simply leaving the house at unusual times, and getting
back home safely, this need not be a problem.

The sort of scenario where the GP, relatives, home carers and the
man who runs the post office collude to overdramatize the risks,
is very common. The 'coroner's court' threat may be levelled at
the social worker: 'If the person with dementia gets lost, or is
attacked by a mugger, or freezes to death, or causes a car
accident, are you prepared to stand up in the coroner's court and
hear the doctor/police officer say, "I strongly advised that s/he
be moved into care, and you refused to consider this course of
action"?'

The following case illustrates the type of situation which
social workers have to deal with, where members of the
community who are disturbed by the 'odd' behaviour of a
neighbour will try to put pressure on the social worker to remove
the person, against their will and their best interests, into
long-term care. It is possible for a social worker who has the
right kind of support to stand firm against this type of pressure
and act as guardian of the client's civil rights, but social workers
often find themselves alone in taking on this role.

## Case study 4

Miss Kempston had lived for 25 years in the same village. She had no family, and was a well-known local personality. Although her short-term memory was poor, she was a good cook and baked cakes regularly. For many years she had attended daily Mass at the Catholic Church in the nearby town where she was well known and liked. She became confused about time, which meant that she sometimes arrived for Mass at unusual times, but the priest managed to deal with this situation.

Initially she refused on more than one occasion to let the social worker in because she did not know her, always talking to her outside the house. The two gradually formed a relationship, and eventually the social worker was invited inside. Miss Kempston began to look forward to the social worker's visits.

Unfortunately, Miss Kempston's neighbours felt that she posed a risk to them as well as to herself, and mounted a vigorous campaign to have her removed into a residential home. Miss Kempston did not wish to move. Her social worker, having completed a risk assessment, agreed that it was not appropriate. Miss Kempston complied with a care package as far as she was able. The risk assessment showed that the description of 'wandering' was inaccurate. She used a familiar taxi company to take her into town and she always found her way home, eventually, after her journeys around the village.

However, there was a risk of fire, as Miss Kempston often forgot to turn off the gas rings on the cooker. The social worker had a smoke detector installed. Unfortunately, the neighbours used this as part of their campaign. They called the fire brigade every time the smoke alarm went off – even if it was only burning toast.

### Case study 4 (continued)

They also made frequent calls to the police. The emergency services were called out so often that a senior police officer contacted the social worker to complain. Fortunately the social worker was a member of a specialist team, well supported by her colleagues. She did not cave in under pressure. The home care package was increased. A tap was fitted to the cooker to control the supply. Miss Kempston formed a close relationship with her home carer and, in time, accepted residential respite care. She remained at home for another two years, as she wanted.

To a social worker in a generic team, lacking both dementia-specific knowledge and the support of colleagues who share specialist experience, this scenario could be very alarming; the social worker's stress might well escalate to a high level. This case clearly illustrates the ageism which is so deeply embedded in the indigenous culture of the United Kingdom. This is often shown in subtle ways, which seem to express concern for the old person.

> There are sometimes 'well-meaning' neighbours, relations and others who appear to think that someone who is old and mentally ill does not have similar needs and feelings in most respects to 'normal' people. When an older person gets labelled mentally ill, there may be an assumption by neighbours that the individual must need continuous protection from the everyday risks which are inherent in living with some degree of independence in the community. Such paternalism, though probably well-intentioned, may be excessive and too restricting of freedom. (Slater and Gearing 1998, p.29)

## The value of a formal risk assessment

In some situations where the social worker has identified that the risk is high, this can be an effective aid to good practice. Local authorities will differ as to whether it always forms part of the initial assessment or not, and social workers will obviously work within the policy of their own department. If it does not form a standard part of the assessment, conducting a formal risk assessment can be a useful tool for the social worker. The identification of the hazards in the person's home or life style which may constitute risk is a useful exercise in clarification.

It is important when assessing all people with dementia, but it is vital where the person lives alone. It is essential that a proper risk assessment be carried out, outlining the hazards, and the probable frequency of hazardous activity taking place. This should be done for others involved in the situation as well as the person with dementia. The social worker is required to assess the risks and manage them to the best of her/his ability. The information should be well documented and placed on the case file so that others may see the process by which the social worker reached the decision.

---

### Case study 5

Mrs Clifton had lived all her life in a small village. Her family had worked on the land for generations. She was used to an outdoor life. She loved to walk over to visit her husband's grave in a churchyard two miles away. As she became disorientated about where she was because of her dementia, she began to get lost. There were several episodes when she went missing and was picked up by the police to be returned to her cottage and her family. Unfortunately for Mrs Clifton, she lived very near to the A1. The risk to other people as well as herself if she walked onto the road was too high to be acceptable.

There is no such thing as a risk-free environment for anyone, of any age. The fact that we feel we should be able to create such an environment for a person with dementia, especially one who lives alone, is rarely questioned. Often the people close to the person with dementia are particularly insistent that he or she must be protected from all danger – even if their quality of life is severely impaired in the process.

If the social worker carries out a full risk assessment in consultation with colleagues and with the family (if there is one), and it is properly documented, it has two functions:

1.  It protects the person with dementia by minimizing the risks.

2.  It reduces stress on the social worker, because it will demonstrate that s/he is aware of the risks and has weighed them up, balancing risk with quality of life.

Supporting people with dementia to live the closing chapters of their lives safely and in a way which affirms their dignity and individuality and is congruent with the way they have chosen to lead their lives in the past is a challenge to both family carers and workers. (Baragwanath 1997, p.106)

The following list outlines some of the factors which can be described as hazards, and which are of particular relevance to the person with dementia. Some or all of them may be relevant to the person who is being assessed. The social worker might use this list of thought-starters when conducting a risk assessment:

1.  the lack of insight and awareness which leads the person to believe that they are perfectly safe

2.  the possibility of catastrophic reactions being caused by triggers in the environment, such as specific things which other people say or do

3.     issues associated with transport, such as refusing
       to fasten the seat-belt, or trying to leave a moving
       vehicle

4.     dietary issues – malnutrition, not being able to
       maintain diets needed for medical conditions,
       overeating

5.     medication – either forgetting to take it, or risking
       an overdose of prescribed or non-prescription drugs

6.     the difficulty of obtaining informed consent to a
       variety of procedures

7.     problems with spatial awareness leading to a fall
       caused, for example, by missing the seats of chairs, or
       misperceiving of the size of steps, etc.

8.     distortion of perception leading to hallucinations
       and delusions

9.     problems with communication

10.    the inability to comply with instructions, such as
       in the use of physiotherapy aids.

Each of these hazards should be assessed to estimate the degree
of risk presented by each. It is important that risk assessments, as
well as care plans, should be passed over to the out-of-hours
emergency duty team if somebody has been assessed as 'high
risk'. Having done that, the social worker should be able to leave
the workplace, knowing that all reasonable steps have been
taken. If something goes then disastrously wrong the social
worker is not compromised. The social worker is required to
assess the risk, take all reasonable steps to minimize hazards, and
to monitor the situation. S/he has then discharged the duty of
care. The social worker is not required to see that the client never
comes to any harm. This is clearly impossible.

## ELDER ABUSE

Social workers who practise in this field are aware that a person with dementia is particularly vulnerable to various kinds of abuse. It can be physical, psychological or emotional. It can involve negligence or financial and sexual exploitation.

A person with dementia may forget the details of what has happened. They may be unable to tell others what has happened to them, and if they do tell someone else there is a good chance that they will not be believed. Abusers are obviously aware of the situation. In this sense a person with dementia is in the same situation as a child. It is a power situation in which the person with dementia, like the child, is almost totally lacking in power.

Local authority social services departments are required to have a policy on elder abuse, and social workers who work with people with dementia will obviously be aware of their local guidelines and the line management chain and procedures to be followed if abuse is suspected.

The question of elder abuse is very complex and difficult to work with, and different local authorities have used different definitions. There is no consensus about a definition of abuse in older people, although there is agreement that it takes different forms. It may be helpful to start from the position that older people have rights, and that abuse occurs when a person is deprived of a satisfactory quality of life. These rights have been listed as: 'the right to choose, the right to privacy, the right to independence, the right to a decent quality of life and the right to protection and safety' (Pritchard 1992, p.25). Although we can all agree that these rights exist, the problem of how they are interpreted is very subjective and will be changed by the age, social class and ethnicity of the individuals concerned.

Social workers will be aware that people with dementia are at risk of abuse of all kinds from other people. But it is also true that people with dementia abuse their carers, as the following case illustrates.

## Case example 6

Bill and Sarah Turvey had been married for over sixty years. Sarah was eighty-two and her husband, who had been suffering from Alzheimer's disease for five years, was two years older. Bill was a big man who had been a boxer in his youth. He had started to visit the day centre, which he seemed to enjoy. When he could no longer attend to his own personal hygiene he became very frustrated and directed his anger at his wife. One day he grabbed her by the wrist and held her arm under the hot tap when she was running his bath, and she was unable to persuade him to let her go. After this incident both Bill and Sarah were extremely upset and Bill was remorseful, saying that he would never do it again. But, after a visit to the doctor, Sarah contacted her social worker in some distress. They reassessed the situation and Sarah admitted for the first time that Bill had hit her on two occasions while she was trying to change his clothes in the morning. Sarah also admitted that Bill had always had a short temper and had occasionally 'given her a smack' when they were both much younger.

The case was reassessed and it was agreed that Bill might accept help with personal care more easily from someone other than his wife. A home care package was set up. Fortunately Bill had no difficulty in accepting help with personal care from a home carer, and he was able to stay at home for another year.

Financial abuse is very common, in spite of the existence of the Court of Protection. Unscrupulous relatives, for example, can abuse the enduring power of attorney.

The decision to intervene in situations of abuse should not be taken lightly, since adults do have a right to self-determination. For people with dementia this is no different. Professionals must decide how to maintain the balance between protection of the individual and the rights of the carer while not colluding with abusive practice or avoiding the situation. (Phair 1997, p.91)

It is hoped that the proposed reform of the law to protect adults who lack mental capacity will help to reduce the amount of abuse. Certainly the present legal system, which depends upon the person who has been abused being able to press charges against their abuser, is clearly inadequate to protect people with dementia.

The area of elder abuse is one where the social worker should consult colleagues as widely as possible and be entitled to support from senior staff in order to be able to offer adequate protection to their clients.

## SUMMARY

- The physical and mental decline which usually accompanies life in the seventh, eighth and ninth decades has certain features which affect everyone. However, people with dementia have special needs which demand specialist expertise.

- The assessment of people with dementia also requires special skills because of the specific problems which it presents. These include problems which may arise, such as difficulty in making the initial contact with the person, achieving the balance between the person's right to autonomy and their need for help, and their need for emotional support throughout the process.

- Care planning with people with dementia includes addressing the challenge of encouraging and helping them and their families to accept services. Care plans need constant readjustment.

- Risk is an important issue which social workers have to address. Conducting a full risk assessment is valuable.

- The issue of elder abuse requires attention in relation to people with dementia.

# CHAPTER FIVE

# The Emotional and Social World of the Person with Dementia

## INTRODUCTION

The purpose of this chapter is to highlight the emotional and social world of people with dementia and their families. Powerful emotions, taken in conjunction with the way that people relate to each other, form the social context in which families experiencing dementia function. Two theoretical approaches emphasizing the importance of the emotional and social world in understanding dementia are described:

- Attachment theory gives us a model for understanding the behaviour of individuals who find themselves in a situation of prolonged uncertainty.

- Systems theory gives us a model for understanding the family as a system which governs itself according to its own rules, the behaviour of individuals within the family affecting, and being affected by, the behaviour of other members of the system.

This topic leads us to examine the question of whether the needs of these emotional/social systems can be met within the current framework of care management with older people.

## THE IMPORTANCE OF EMOTION

In order to improve practice, social workers in this field have to learn more about the emotional needs of everyone involved in the situation, including their own. It is not only people with dementia who behave in apparently incomprehensible ways. Carers, too, can exhibit behaviour which seems to be irrational and incomprehensible to those who are not able to understand their emotional reality.

The case example of the Carlton family which was introduced in Chapter Four (p.75 ) serves to illustrate the importance of working with the emotional currents in a family. At the point where the social worker became involved with this family there were several areas of conflict – some new and some of long standing. If these were not addressed, it would be difficult to make sensible decisions.

Good practice indicates that in this type of situation the social worker should meet with all the family, in the absence of their mother. A family meeting should be convened. It does not need to be a case conference with all the quasi-legal issues which that implies. If possible the social worker should ask a colleague to be present if the family is large and emotions are likely to run high. There is a dual purpose for such a meeting. First, it provides a forum in which the family can ventilate their emotions in a safe environment. In this part of the meeting the social worker is acting as a facilitator. In the latter part of the meeting the social worker can then, using her/his care management skills, help the family to make the decisions which urgently need to be made, instead of arguing with each other.

In the case of the Carlton family the issue of the sale of the house, if residential care is chosen as the preferred option, would

## Case Example 7 – the Carlton family story continued

The situation had been made more difficult by the fact that Mr Carlton had decided not to share with his children the fact that his wife had become seriously mentally impaired.

None of the children felt particularly close to their mother. She had always been a hypochondriac (or semi-invalid) who was unable to meet their needs for parenting. It was their father who, they all felt, showed them the love and care they needed when they were growing up. His death acted as a catalyst on the family, reopening old wounds.

Ann, as the only daughter, had assumed the role of 'main carer', trying to be 'housewife, mum and superstar', until her own emotional and physical health suffered and the quality of her own family life was undermined. She had a closer relationship with her mother than her brothers did, but she was very worried at the time about her eldest daughter who was showing signs of depression.

Peter accepted responsibility for a clearly defined and limited role, refusing to step outside it. He accepted full responsibility for his mother's finances but ignored her needs for hands-on care. He refused to engage with the powerful feelings of loss and grief which followed his father's death, or the feelings of loss, guilt and resentment caused by the discovery of his mother's extreme dependency.

Richard, the youngest child, had suffered most from the effect of his mother's ill health when he was young. He had resented her inability to mother him all his adult life. Now he was grieving bitterly for his father. He was totally unable to accept that his mother was suffering from Alzheimer's disease. He showed no reaction to the news at all. The fact that he lived a hundred miles away made it possible for him to opt out completely.

## Case Example 7 – the Carlton family story continued

Richard and Peter had been close as children, but a serious dispute between them had started ten years before when a substantial loan from Peter to Richard was never repaid.

David, seeing his wife Ann becoming depressed and ill, was feeling extremely angry with her brothers for allowing her to shoulder the whole burden of caring for their mother. He himself had offered little in the way of practical support, and felt guilty about this when she collapsed.

At this point Richard and Peter unexpectedly made an alliance against David. They both felt strongly that their mother should remain in the family home, as they needed the money which they expected to inherit when the house was sold. However, they had not considered how this was to be achieved.

It was at this difficult and delicate stage in the life of the Carlton family that the social worker had to enter the scene. Clearly decisions about Mrs Carlton's future had to be made quickly.

have to be addressed. The family would have to grasp the nettle and talk about the family finances, either in the meeting or separately, without the social worker present.

Obviously it would not be appropriate for Mrs Carlton herself to be present at such a meeting. This is an example of a situation where good practice for decision-making is different in the case of older, physically frail and mentally able people, and of older people with dementia. Mrs Carlton at present has not the power, if she ever had it, to defend herself against the great force of her children's emotions, which are likely to appear to her as an attack. Even if she is not present, it is likely that one of the children, possibly Ann, will feel impelled to act as a strong advocate for her mother's rights.

A serious attempt must be made to find out what Mrs Carlton wants to do at this point. She might find it easier to talk to the social worker with none of the family present, or she may select one of her children to act as her supporter and advocate. Or there might be someone else who could fill this role – a friend or neighbour.

Our emotional lives are crucially important to all of us. The social worker must be able to engage with the underlying emotions of all the parties concerned if needed – emotions which are often very powerful. This is an area in which social workers who were trained in Rogerian counselling techniques would have felt confident and competent. However, care management for older people with dementia, with its present emphasis on assessment and planning rather than counselling, has meant that some skills have been lost, making the social work task harder and more stressful than it used to be.

Experience would suggest that unless the emotions of clients are taken fully into account, an accurate assessment of need cannot be made, nor can a care package be developed which will be really acceptable to the client and/or the carer. Unfortunately, it is not something which can be quickly learned. There is no 'quick fix'.

It is helpful to clarify the situation by looking separately at the two groups of people.

## The emotional needs of the person with dementia

We now have a better understanding of what the emotional needs of people with dementia are, thanks to the work of two leading social psychologists working in the field, notably Bere Miesen and the late Tom Kitwood. Kitwood laid out a framework of these needs saying that

> it may be helpful to think of five great needs which overlap, coming together in the central need for love: comfort, attachment, inclusion, occupation and identity. The fulfilment of one of these needs will, to some extent, involve the fulfilment of the others. (Kitwood 1997, p.81)

The person-centred approach tells us that the behaviour of a person with dementia, which is perceived by others as 'difficult' or 'challenging', is often an attempt to communicate emotions. Miesen (1997), commenting on the chapter by Droes, concludes that

> Her overview (of the psychosocial approaches) confirms the increasing trend of researchers and clinicians to try to move into the dementia sufferer's inner world: to understand their feelings, experiences and manner of coping with a disease they never asked for. Apparently meaningless behaviour, on closer examination, is full of meaning. (Miesen 1997, p.342)

Staff of many of the organizations which provide residential and day care now understand that they need to learn about this inner world of people with dementia. Various techniques such as the use of reminiscence, life-story work, music, drama and poetry, and the use of sensory therapies are all being used in this country and others as ways to enter the world of the person with dementia and communicate with them. Information about innovations and techniques which have been tried and trusted for several years is available in journals such as the *Journal of Dementia Care*. (Details can be found in at the end of this book.)

## Finding out what the person with dementia wants

Many people with dementia have problems with communication through speech. They may start a sentence and be unable to finish it, or they may be unable to find the words to express what they want to say. They may not know what they want to say. All this leads them to feel isolated and can drive them further down into despair.

However, skills for communicating more effectively with people with dementia can be learned. This is not easy. Malcolm Goldsmith says

> The responsibility for easing the communication process must be ours. It is a skilled job and we will need a great deal of patience. Perhaps we should approach it as though learning a foreign language – some people seem to be naturally gifted and born linguists and a new language seems to come easily to them, but everyone has to work at it. Similarly when we are with people with dementia, to hear their voice may be quite a challenge. It may tax us intellectually and stretch our imagination. It will test our patience and it will bring surprises and setbacks but also moments of clarity which make it all worthwhile. (Goldsmith 1997, p.24)

This expertise is now available to be shared – but it is being used almost exclusively within the provider section of the social care service. It is providers of day care and residential and nursing care who are beginning to gain expertise in this area.

However, if an empathetic bond is created, imaginative guesswork based on what the social worker knows of the person's past life and present circumstances should help.

We already know something about what a person with dementia does not want, through working with people in long-term care settings: they do not want to be treated as children. This means that they do not want to be ignored, talked about behind their backs, or expected to complete tasks at a speed which they can no longer manage – tasks which they could complete successfully if given enough time.

All the 'personal detractions' identified (Kitwood 1997, p.46) as part of the 'malignant social psychology' in long-term care can also be found in the lives of many people who are living at home. They occur in the context of interactions between the person and the family, partner and friends, or between the person and the doctor, or the psychiatrist, or the social worker, or the community psychiatric nurse or the home care worker.

The loss of a sense of identity which comes with the loss of memory of your past life means that your identity has to be held in trust for you by other people. Your sense of connectedness to other people, to the community and to the greater reality of the world is also seriously threatened by memory loss.

The self-esteem of people with dementia is very fragile and the fact that they often find themselves in a situation where it is further undermined is a fact of their lives. Many carers, through ignorance, seem to revert to 'parent' mode when dealing with a relative who has poor memory and impaired insight. This is conveyed to the person with dementia by their tone of voice, their body language and the way in which they talk to professionals in the presence of the person, as if they were not there.

We wonder what the person with dementia who is living at home wants, as they are unable to tell us, except obliquely. There is now evidence that people in the early stages of dementia, aware that something is wrong, adopt strategies to adjust to this situation. John Keady has commented upon behaviour he observed in people with dementia.

> For the individual concerned it became vitally important to act upon the suspicions that something was quite seriously wrong and it is usually at this point where *deliberate* action was taken to preserve the self. This was achieved by deploying the tactic of 'closing down' in order to 'construct a new me' from within a cumulative experience of loss. The tactic of closing down emerged as being private and secretive in nature, and was extremely distressing for those close to the individual as they remained completely in the dark over its real purpose and function. (Keady 1997, p.28)

We can also find out what is important to people with dementia by talking to residents in long-term care homes whose dementia tends to be further advanced than it is in those living at home. It is clear from such contacts that the personal, emotional and social aspects of their lives are important to these people. They may have a particular possession which acts both as a talisman and as a cue to who they are and where they come from. But, generally speaking, possessions, money, status and career success cease to have the significance they had before. People with dementia are travelling light. They have no choice but to do so. When they say they want to go home or stay at home, they may or may not be referring to the place where they are living now. 'Home' may be a childhood home or the first home they had when they married. It is a metaphor for happiness, belonging, feeling safe and being able to do what you want. It is as powerful a metaphor as the word 'mother' – a word we so often hear on the lips of people with dementia. It has the same powerful connotations.

Above all, of course, these people want to be as they were before dementia robbed them of their ability to be in control of their own life. This last is a dream which cannot come true. But we can do something to help them feel safe and to enhance their self-esteem, rather than undermine it further.

Social workers are well placed to direct carers to where training in person-centred care is available locally, so that they may learn how to avoid interacting with the person they care for in a way that further damage their self-esteem. If none is available locally social workers should remember that social services are the most powerful purchasers of care services in any area, and should put pressure on their managers to commission such services.

Social workers also have a role to play in ensuring that other professionals in the multidisciplinary team are approaching the person with dementia as well as the carer in a person-centred way. This is an area in which social workers find a particular challenge because of the professional 'pecking-order' in which they find themselves. Social workers feel that their place within the medical hierarchy is often near the bottom. Much educational work still needs to be done in the medical profession and the professions associated with medicine to change attitudes so that everyone adopts the person-centred approach.

The person with dementia as well as the carer may need the services of an advocate – a person who possesses the necessary specialist skills to interpret the needs of the person with dementia and represent them to other professionals. Traditionally this was part of the social work role, and in some circumstances this is still a practical way of working.

## Advocacy

As the role of the social worker has changed under care management, it has become apparent that the advocacy role may sometimes need to be carried out by independent advocates. (This is particularly so where the wishes of the person with dementia conflict with those of the statutory authorities.) An advocate is a person who pleads a cause on behalf of another and generally takes such action as may be necessary to ensure their needs are met and their legal rights are safeguarded. Advocacy can take many different forms, including self-advocacy, lay or citizen advocacy, professional advocacy and collective advocacy.

There are four key reasons why people with dementia need advocates:

- To protect them from physical, emotional and financial abuse.

- To help them make decisions at transitional points in their lives.

- To ensure that their legal rights and entitlements are observed.

- To make sure that they receive a high quality of service and that their individual wishes and preferences are respected as far as possible. (Killeen 1996, p.11)

Advocacy services for people with dementia are still not well developed. There is a need for more pilot services and sensitive evaluation of these services.

Further discussion is needed on the difficult question of advocacy for those who are incapable or unwilling to appoint advocates but are seen to be in need of advocacy.

It is an ethical issue whether individuals who are unable to indicate whether or not they want an advocate should have someone appointed. It leaves the person with dementia very much in the power of the advocate, who at best may find themselves trying to guess what the person might want for themselves and at worst may use the person to fulfil their own agenda. Alternatively, it may be argued that it is morally wrong to pass over someone who is vulnerable and apparently unable to agree to the appointment of an advocate but whose quality of life might be vastly improved by the attention of such a person. (Killeen 1996, p.32)

One of the pilot schemes, which appear to be operating successfully, is the Westminster Advocacy Service for Senior Residents (WASSR), which has established a two-year pilot project for working with people with dementia. The scheme employs the citizen advocacy mode – using a trained volunteer who develops a relationship with their partner/client and stands alongside them, speaking up for their rights. Training is given using person-centred principles. Clients of the scheme are in continuing care at present, but the organizers recognize the need to focus on ways of taking the service to people living in their own homes. WASSR has drawn up a Bill of Rights for People with Dementia, which can be obtained from the scheme and was published in the *Journal of Dementia Care* (Goodchild 1999). This sort of scheme represents an encouraging start.

## The emotional needs of the carer

As I have said, relationships between the person with dementia and their family and friends, and between different members of the family network, often seem to be complicated and difficult for an outsider to comprehend.

Professionals working in the community need to be aware of the importance of the emotional reality of those who are caring for the person in the community. There is one feature of the experience of caring for a person with dementia, which often makes it uniquely painful for some people. It is

> the imperceptibility of the loss. This imperceptibility, which makes the loss of a demented loved person a peculiar loss, is especially unfavourable for the grieving process. In some ways this loss resembles the case of a loved, missing person. This turns the family situation into a chronic, vague, unsafe, emotional arena. (Miesen 1997, p.74)

It is my belief that the failure of social workers to understand and work with the emotional story of the family explains a phenomenon which is a common occurrence to social workers in this field. A care package is created following a needs assessment and is initially accepted by the carer, but then seems never to be quite satisfactory. Different reasons are given why the services which have been accepted are not being used, the days at the day centre are wrong, the home carers are not calling at the right time, the person is refusing to comply, the person has a cold, a sore throat, the carer had a bad night. While we know that small issues can loom very large for carers who are probably physically and emotionally exhausted, there comes a point when the social worker begins to realize that the care package is being sabotaged.

Closer investigation of the family dynamics would probably reveal that there is often considerable emotion within the family, which the social worker has not attempted to uncover. Guilt can be an overwhelming emotion for family members. Or the problem may be that not all the family can accept the diagnosis, or that important members of the family system are struggling with extremely powerful negative emotions which make it very hard for them to make rational decisions. 'Deathbed' promises made to one dying parent that the children will never 'put the other parent in a home' can further complicate the situation.

The social worker might also have made the elementary mistake of only talking to one member of the family about the situation, without checking to see how the other members felt. Often it is the family member with a strongly held view who talks to the social worker first to make their views known. He or she may believe that the person must move into long-term care within the next few days. Or the carer, while telling the social worker that the situation is completely impossible and that they cannot continue like this, will systematically refuse all community care services which are offered. It is only later that other family members will contact the social worker often with a completely different view of the problem.

In some situations the social worker can do nothing but wait for the crisis to develop before the family will feel able to accept help. This is hard on the social worker, who may feel guilty that s/he is not doing anything to help, but it may be the only course of action to follow. Families have a right to refuse services. They also have a right to change their minds. The social worker has to learn to distinguish  between a rational decision to refuse help and emotionally driven sabotage.

Another phenomenon which occurs quite often is that a family, having supported a partner and parent for some considerable time with a good care package, seems to need to create a crisis in order to give themselves permission to say that they can no longer continue to provide care at home. This often seems to occur in large families with several adult children who started out on the journey through care by saying that they would never allow their parent to 'go into a home'. The social worker will be able to help these families by telling them that very few families indeed do manage to care for the relative with dementia until the end of their life, and that when the point has been reached where the person needs twenty-four-hour care, he or she may be better cared for in a long-term care home.

A complicating factor, of course, is that the family home may have to be sold in order to pay for the long-term care. This means that the children will not receive their inheritance. It is not socially acceptable for family members to tell the social worker that this is their reason for keeping an elderly parent at home when they manifestly are unable to cope. Therefore, all sorts of reasons are given to the social worker by the family in order to explain why they have decided to keep the person at home. The financial assessment should be completed as soon as possible after the initial contact has been made, for this reason. The social worker will know then what s/he is dealing with and can proceed accordingly.

Sometimes these tensions within families have little or nothing to do with the dementia of the spouse, partner or parent. Family conflicts which predate the dementia by many years influence how the family responds to their relative's dementia. In some instances the parties who are in conflict would be better off apart. It is also true that many carers in these situations are so exhausted and stressed by the task of providing one-to-one care on a twenty-four-hour basis that they do not know themselves what they want or what they need.

## It is the carer who decides how much help the person with dementia receives

The social worker should always be aware that it is actually the carer who decides how much respite is needed, how many days a week their relative should attend the day centre, how much residential respite care the person has. In reality, the carer's needs often predominate over the needs of the person with dementia. This relationship is one in which power is a significant factor, and the power scales are clearly weighted in favour of the person who has the capacity to tell the professionals how they feel and what their needs are.

There are partners and families who want the person with dementia to be taken into long-term care even when they could be maintained at home with a community care package. In these situations it may be clear that the person with dementia wants to stay at home and would be able to do so with support services, but they will not be allowed to. They might in fact be better off at this point in their lives if they were on their own without a partner. Social workers are often very conscious of this but they have to be pragmatic.

This is one of the difficult tensions which form an integral part of the job of the social worker in this field, and it can be very difficult to accept. The reform of the law to protect adults who lack mental capacity may strengthen the social worker as s/he tries to find out what the person with dementia wants and how they feel. However it is hard for the social worker to maintain a person at home with community care support if the family does not want this to happen. The person with no family is, para-doxically, more likely to remain living in the community, provided they can be persuaded to accept help.

The duty to presume that the person does possess mental capacity unless proved otherwise should improve such situations and ensure that civil rights are not eroded (Lord Chancellor's Office 1997a).

## Anti-discriminatory practice

All social workers will be aware of the hierarchies which exist within our society, and clearly older people who suffer from mental impairment are going to find their place near the bottom of any hierarchy. If these people are also women, and if they are in addition black, they will be right at the bottom of the pile. They are the victims of 'multiple oppression'. This concept is developed by Neil Thompson:

> oppression and discrimination are presented as aspects of the divisive nature of social structure – reflections of the social divisions of class, race, gender, age, disability and sexual orientation. These are dimensions of our social location and so we need to understand them as a whole – as facets of an overall edifice of power and dominance rather than separate or discreet entities. (Thompson 1993, p.11)

Work with this client group has always reflected this lack of status within society at large, a fact of which social workers in the field are surely aware. The discrimination which exists within families against the older person with dementia is often very obvious. However, the area is extremely complex. How does the social worker balance the rights of a middle-aged woman who feels she has a right to a life of her own after years of child-rearing and does not want to care for her mother at home against the rights of the old woman with dementia who wants to remain in the bosom of her daughter's family? It is an impossible choice. Fortunately, the choice is not for the social worker to make. The family will make the decision and the social worker's task is to support all the family members as they make it.

## THE VALUE OF A THEORETICAL FRAMEWORK

The social worker who is working in this field needs to have particular skills in this area. Many social workers will find it helpful to have a theoretical framework which explains the behaviours which they commonly observe in the families with whom they are working. Having found this to be useful myself, I include below a brief examination of two such theories which helped me to understand the behaviour of the people with whom I was working.

There are a great many theories put forward to explain the behaviour of people with dementia. The following discussion pertains to two theories which rely on emotion to explain behaviour, both in the person with dementia and their carers.

## Attachment theory

A theory of human behaviour which appears to have particular relevance to our client group is that of 'attachment'. This is a theoretical framework which helps the social worker to gain a better understanding of the underlying dynamics of the relevant relationships. An understanding of the long-standing attachment needs of both the carer and the person with dementia is invaluable to guiding people in their journey through care. The social worker will find it helpful to be reminded of the importance of attachment theory.

Bowlby, in his seminal work with children in the decades following the last war, developed the theory of attachment. He defined attachment behaviour as 'behaviour that has proximity to an attachment figure as a predictable outcome and whose elementary function is protection of the infant from danger'. (Bowlby 1969, cited in Goldburg *et al.* 1995, p.63) He showed that small children display a powerful need to be physically close to their primary attachment figure (usually but not always the mother) in order to feel safe. 'The infant and young child should experience a warm, intimate and continuous relationship with his mother (or permanent mother substitute) in which both find satisfaction and enjoyment' (Bowlby 1951, p.51).

The classic trigger for attachment behaviour is a feeling of danger. Bowlby identified three types of separation response: protest, despair and denial. From these emotional responses he named two broad categories of response to separation: secure and insecure. Securely attached infants would demonstrate distress on separation but could be comforted by others, or by the mother on her return. The insecurely attached infants were inconsolable and took longer to calm down. Later Bowlby and others expanded the theory of attachment.

Ainsworth and Wittig developed the 'strange situation' experiment in Baltimore in 1969. In this experiment the infant was separated from the mother for a short period and observed closely under experimental conditions during the separation and during the reunion with the mother. Securely attached infants were distressed by the separation but could be consoled. Insecurely attached infants, however, had a different response:

> A few of the one-year olds from the Baltimore study were surprisingly angry when the mother returned after a three-minute (or shorter) separation. They cried and wanted contact but would not simply cuddle or 'sink in' when picked up by the returning mother; they showed their ambivalence by kicking or swiping at her. Another group of children seemed to snub or avoid the mother on reunion, even though they had often searched for her while she was gone. (Bretherton 1995, p.61)

A crucial point about attachment behaviour is that, once triggered, all other activities stop until proximity with the attachment figure is achieved. The interesting factor which these psychologists were able to demonstrate was that these patterns of attachment behaviour are fixed by the end of infancy and become internalized as part of the personality. They demonstrated this through follow-up experiments with the infants in the Ainsworth study until they reached the age of seventeen.

> Between infancy and adulthood lies a process of development whereby the adult no longer needs physical proximity to an attachment figure to feel safe. Experience enables a person to understand what is happening, to contain emotional reactions and to work out what needs to be done... The need for physical closeness does not disappear

> altogether in adult life. It remains for most people as a regular part of intimate relationships, and faced with stress, many adults take comfort from physical proximity to a trusted person. However, this need for closeness does not have the urgency of infancy. Adults can wait, whereas in infants, all exploration and play is halted until proximity is achieved. (Bruce 1998, p.193)

People develop individual styles of attachment behaviour, which persist throughout life.

We now know, through the work of Bere Miesen and others who have built upon Bowlby's original work, that persons with dementia repeatedly find themselves in 'a strange situation'. The internal models which people have developed in order to cope with separation anxiety no longer work for people with dementia because they are highly cognitive, and cognition, as we know, is affected by dementia.

Miesen puts forward the theory that

> remaining aware of one's cognitive dysfunctioning in dementia is like going into a 'strange situation' in which the person experiences feeling unsafe for long periods of time, powerless and with no structures to hold onto' (Miesen 1997, p.68).

The carer very often becomes the attachment figure, and this explains the well-known phenomenon of the carer who cannot leave the person at all without provoking extreme distress. The extent to which this type of behaviour occurs probably relates to the attachment needs and history of the person with dementia and of the carer:

> While there are clearly relevant differences in caring for a person with dementia who is an adult and has experienced independence, attachment theory suggests that our experiences of parenting shape the ways in which we negotiate caregiving and care receiving in relationships throughout life. (Bruce 1998, p.199)

## Respite care and attachment behaviour

Respite may provoke extreme separation anxiety and add more 'strangeness' to the everyday experience of dementia, which is itself, for many people, a 'strange situation'. This often provokes attachment behaviour such as clinging to the carer, refusing to go, searching, calling and refusing to settle while away from home. 'Punishment' responses, such as angry or rejecting behaviour, can be shown towards the carer when they are reunited. These behaviours can make carers feel that the price of the break is too high. What they have to go through before and/or after a respite, in addition to their anxiety about how the person with dementia is feeling while away from them, may seem too much to bear. So social workers need to be aware that carers, as well as people with dementia, may equally show separation anxiety under these circumstances.

The way the carer responds will depend in some degree upon their own attachment history. The social worker needs to understand these apparently irrational responses to the offer of respite care, and to support both parties through the process so that both may benefit. The attachment theory paradigm does explain the behaviour of the carer who refuses to accept any help which involves separation from the person with dementia, even though they are clearly approaching 'burn-out' through physical and emotional exhaustion.

Attachment needs are extremely powerful emotional drivers, which lead people to make emotional rather than rational decisions. If the social worker fails to take this into account much effort, time (and therefore money) will be wasted by the professionals in the field who are setting up care packages. However, as has been pointed out, with careful handling of the situation, which includes preparation of the carer and the person with dementia about what to expect, and prior advice and information to the carer about how best to handle the situation, the residential respite service can be extremely beneficial. It needs to be offered in as flexible a way as possible. The carer should be able to have a break of two or three nights or maybe even two or three weeks. The social worker needs to be aware, however, that respite care is of real benefit to the carer in the short term.

> Relief care gave them (the carers) the opportunity to rest and recuperate, to have free evenings and week-ends, to have a holiday, to devote more time to other relatives and friends, and to maintain their homes. (Levin *et al.* 1994, p.164)

It enables the person with dementia to remain living at home longer by giving the carer a rest, and therefore the person with dementia will benefit in the long run – although the carer may not particularly enjoy sending them to respite care in the short term, at least initially.

For many people with dementia who still possess insight, the fact that the carer needs a break can be an acceptable reason for persuading them to agree to a respite short stay. As has already been stated, the social worker should be aware, and should warn the carer, that the person will be more confused after a short stay. There are two possible reasons for this. It may be because the person is confused and disorientated after a period of time in a strange place. Or s/he may be showing one of the classic attachment responses to reunion following separation, by punishing the attachment figure.

## Systems theory

The second theory which I have found to be of assistance to the social worker in this field is systems theory in its practical application. This approach has been used within childcare for some time, but has only entered the field of social work with older people in recent years. The theory states that

> families are socially constructed units, based upon relationships of kinship, obligation and intimacy which exert a powerful socializing influence on the behaviour and understanding of their members ... the worker using a

family therapy approach will view the individual's 'symptom' as part of an interactional pattern and herself as a facilitator, enabling the family to harness its own strengths and flexibility towards a solution. (White 1997, p.185)

The dementia process can generate considerable family stress because of the many problems which arise within a short space of time, and the many decisions which may have to be made on behalf of the person with dementia. The decisions can be so many and so complex that they can bring the family into a dysfunctional state. 'Dementia is an illness which generally impacts on the whole family and it is therefore valuable for workers in this field to develop skills in intervening with the family as a unit' (Sherlock and Gardner 1993, p.63)

The theoretical approach is clearly attractive to the social worker in this field who has to work with family groups of adults who are often showing high levels of expressed emotion:

A central discourse within family therapy, is how best to share power with families in a way which allows them to take responsibility for their own choices but retains safety for all members. Power should be reframed as the responsibility to create a safe environment within which the family can find its own solutions. The worker should use her expertise in systems theory and family relationships to work alongside the family, help them to make sense of their world, and explore differences and alternatives available to them. (White 1997, p.189)

Alison Roper-Hall is a pioneer in the field of developing systemic therapy with older adults and has written extensively on the subject. Among many other topics, she discusses the challenges which are implicit in developing a working relationship with an older person. She asks, 'How will a referred adult view being seen with other family members? How easy will it be for family members to attend? Who should be invited and how is this explained to the older adult referred?' She quotes the example of a man in his seventies 'who came for a first family therapy appointment, not knowing what to expect, [and] said in amazement and disbelief, "You mean just talking about it can make a difference?"' and goes on to write:

> The generations currently aged over 65 years may have less belief than younger people that psychological concepts offer useful ways of understanding their situation. The prevailing cultural metaphors for most of their lives, in Western society at least, have been mechanistic, and ideas of illness have been met with expectations of treatment within a medical model. (Roper-Hall 1993, p.194)

There is a clear problem here in finding space and time to practice as a systemic worker within care management, for all the reasons described in this book. However, the approach offers tools such as genograms and ecomaps which can be used quickly and easily by the busy social worker to analyse and understand a family situation. An ecomap – a diagrammatic representation of the family system – can be drawn on a scrap of paper while talking to a client on the phone. A genogram – a simple family tree – can be used in the same way to help the social worker obtain a clear picture from a stressed carer who is trying to describe the family situation. Techniques such as the making of contracts and the use of 'circular questioning' can be useful in family meetings, as well as using the approach as a tool to analyse the dynamics of the meeting.

Both these theoretical approaches can be very useful in assisting social workers in

> obtaining and recording data about the social context of families experiencing dementia. It is expected that this contextualised approach will assist practitioners to 'individualize' care plans, as opposed to issuing a 'standard' care plan. (LeNavenec 1997, p.211)

It is the social context surrounding the dementia which is important for the social worker to understand.

Discussion of these two theories brings us directly to one of the central questions which are posed by this book.

## DOES CARE MANAGEMENT FOR OLDER PEOPLE MEET THE NEEDS OF PEOPLE AND FAMILIES EXPERIENCING DEMENTIA?

I have already referred to the social context of the family experiencing dementia. By this I mean the emotional reality of both the person with dementia and the carer(s) and the family or network system in which those individuals exist. This is the key concept which is missing from the care management model.

The traditional way of working as though there were only one client does not meet the needs of people and families experiencing dementia, as it is not addressing the issue of multiple clients. Nor does it recognise the skill and extra time which are needed to assess the person with dementia. As we have seen, social work for dementia has been bolted on to generic care of older people, which, as we know, was primarily developed for work with people who are physically infirm but mentally capable.

Some situations in this field are extremely complex. Although it is now understood that the needs of carers have to be considered as well as those of the person with dementia, the way data is collected from referral forms by senior managers continues to inform the social worker that the assumption is that the client is a single individual – the person with dementia. The medical model from which this was derived is apparently (and unfortunately) still intact.

When we refer back to the four main care management tasks – the assessment of need, the designing of a care package, and the monitoring and reviewing of that care package (see also page 52) – we can see that they are seen as time-limited, one-off activities, which, once completed, stay completed. That is why social workers are instructed to close cases once the care management task is complete. However, social workers in the field of dementia know that this model simply does not work. The time and effort involved in completing the paperwork and inputting data on the computer to close the case is wasted when the case has to be reopened within a short time. It is interesting that social workers who work with other client groups, particularly with children, do still engage in what the Barclay Report referred to as 'long term work'. Clearly the needs of children are seen as deserving and requiring this approach. It is significant that the 'community care experiment' has not been seen to apply to children. But in the very large number of adult cases, particularly people who are chronically disabled and older people, the care management model has been rigorously followed as community care has been implemented. It has been used as a tool to ration the amount of time spent on each case and so allow the assessment of more new cases.

Families experiencing dementia represent one of the largest groups of people who are experiencing a peculiarly catastrophic loss, which puts the whole family system under strain. Clearly these people are not receiving the service they need from social services or the health care system at present. Their needs are different in degree and in duration from those of other older people. For this reason we may argue that a radical rethink is necessary if their needs are to be met adequately.

Several factors have combined to mean that this group of people is disadvantaged. As a group they usually have both health and social needs. Because they have both it is easy to pass them from one sector to the other, each claiming that they are the responsibility of the other. As we have seen the planners in social services have always found it difficult to decide whether they fall within services for older people, or mental health services. As a result they have often fallen between the two.

The community for which social services are required to provide care has been redefined by the introduction, three years after the NHS and Community Care Act was implemented, of the eligibility criteria. These criteria are currently being used as a means of rationing services by excluding those with low-priority needs. This means that the person with dementia has to be exhibiting extremely disturbed behaviour, and/or the carer has to be at the point of physical and/or emotional collapse, before they qualify for help from social services. This extremely shortsighted policy saves some money in the short term at the cost of an unacceptable level of human misery. Voluntary sector organizations are increasingly being forced to fill this gap in service provision, often at great cost to themselves. On the whole families do not just walk away from their family member who can no longer live independently because of dementia. They will and do carry on until they reach breaking point.

GPs are and always have been the only people who see everyone in the country. So far the annual over-seventy-five checks appear to have had little effect on increasing the diagnosis and treatment rate for dementia. People are not being passed on either to social services or to the voluntary sector for help.

We saw in the case of the Carlton family how ineffective the framework provided by care management is for dealing with a complex family situation. The paperwork generated by computer systems is not nearly sensitive enough to allow for good practice.

Clearly this is an area of work where more resources need to be directed. Specialist training of social workers in dementia and the creation of more specialist teams will inevitably cost money.

As we have already seen, there are 750,000 people with dementia in the UK in the year 2000, and only 17,000 of them are under the age of 65 (Alzheimer's Society, Information Section, January 2000). The cost to the state of caring for them is extremely high. This may explain why, in spite of sustained pressure from groups such as the Alzheimer's Society, no government appears to be prepared to grasp the nettle and publish a comprehensive plan to meet their health and social care needs. It seems paradoxical that the very size of the problem means that a solution cannot be found.

## SUMMARY

- Cognition is affected much earlier in dementia than the emotional activity of the brain. Emotions may, in fact, make up the main reality for people with dementia who are still living at home, and it is very important to understand them. It is possible to learn to communicate with people with dementia.

- Carers are also likely to be struggling to manage a complex mixture of powerful emotions. This means that the social worker in this field must be able to engage with the underlying emotions of all the parties.

- Two theories which explain relevant aspects of human behaviour are examined in this chapter as a means of helping the social worker to understand and therefore work more effectively with people with dementia, and the families and networks to which they belong. These are attachment theory and systems theory. They form the social context of the person, which we must understand if we are to be effective as social workers in this field.

- It is clear that these situations are extremely complex, but it is by no means clear that the care management model is the one best suited to work with this client group. The way that the community for which social services have a duty to provide care has been redefined, and the various obstacles which are still deeply entrenched within the social services system, are briefly discussed in this chapter.

# CHAPTER SIX

# Cultural Difference

## INTRODUCTION

Different individuals, depending on their life history and personality, experience dementia differently. In addition to these personal differences there is a cultural dimension, which determines the response of the person and of those who care for them. In this chapter we shall look at the importance of ethnicity, social class, age and sexual orientation in shaping both the way dementia is experienced and the way services are provided.

It is an undisputed fact that our society contains a rich mix of people of all ages, many different ethnic groups, cultures and lifestyles and it is vital that social workers show genuine awareness of and sensitivity towards this fact. Social workers must be aware of the differentials of power and the potential for oppression which exist within society. An understanding of the theory and the practice of anti-oppressive social work is important for practitioners in the field.

In the case of our client group we are dealing for the most part with old people who suffer from a condition which is commonly classed as a mental illness. The majority of them are women. Clearly it is not helpful to regard them as victims of a specific form of discrimination. A framework for anti-oppressive social work theory and practice is offered by Dalrymple and Burke, who suggest that we use the concept of a dual perspective:

The use of the dual perspective enables us to locate an individual's personal experience of oppression within the context of her or his social environment. It enables us to evaluate our own value position in relation to others and thus to take account of differences and similarities. It helps us to understand powerlessness and through this the nature of power within society. (Dalrymple and Burke 1995, p.21)

Common examples of difference with which social workers in the field of dementia need to be especially familiar are language, ethnicity, social class, age and sexual orientation.

## LANGUAGE

The need to communicate with all people in a language which they understand is now regarded as a matter of importance, and some resources are committed to it by social services departments and health trusts. However, there are simply not enough staff from the ethnic minorities to ensure that people with dementia will always find someone with whom they can converse in their first language. The great number of languages spoken in the UK presents social workers with a daunting task. However, each city, town or village should be aware of the most common languages spoken in the geographical area and a list of interpreters should be available from social services and/or the local health trust.

The practice of using family members to interpret is quite inappropriate and should cease as soon as possible. Relatives will be tempted to say what *they* want to say, putting it into the mouth of the person with dementia. If the person makes very negative statements the relative may feel that s/he cannot interpret them accurately because they are too personal or even abusive. The following example shows how this can happen.

The need for advocates for people with dementia has already been well documented. How much more important is it for people with dementia from the ethnic minority groups?

## Case study 8

Bulwant Singh was over twenty-five years older than his wife Katari Kaur. When he developed dementia their two sons were still at school. Bulwant had spoken English but had forgotten it as the dementia progressed and was now only able to communicate in fragmentary Punjabi – his first language. His wife Katari had never learned English.

They had both come to the town from Pakistan as adults, to join Bulwant's son by his first marriage. Unfortunately the son had moved away. The social worker was asked by the GP, who was also a Sikh, to make an assessment and set up a care package. She spoke no Punjabi so she asked Harminder, a Punjabi-speaking care assistant from the day centre, to go with her to act as interpreter.

Katari had a clear request to put before the social worker. She wanted major adaptation to the house so that a WC and shower could be installed on the ground floor. This was not within the social worker's remit. In discussing this (through Harminder) the social worker felt that Katari was showing considerable negative emotion, so she asked her (through Harminder) how she felt about her husband's illness. When the question was asked Katari burst into tears and replied at length – clearly very distressed. Unfortunately Harminder said that she felt unable to repeat what Katari had said because it would be disrespectful. The social worker had to insist, and learned that Katari was very bitter because she, a woman in her late forties, was stuck looking after a man in his middle seventies. At the same time she had two children in their early teens at home. There was a serious conflict of roles for her because she was the mother of young children as well as the carer of an old person. She was particularly angry that Bulwant's son had moved to a city 100 miles away and they hardly ever saw him. She felt that social services should make him come back and help her to look after his father.

## Case study 8 (continued)

A discussion then took place (again through Harminder) about what help would be acceptable to Katari Kaur – home care, day care, etc. At the conclusion of the visit the social worker felt that it had not gone well and discussed the question of interpretation with Harminder. Harminder explained that as a young woman she felt very embarrassed questioning a woman like Katari, who was older than herself. She was unable to accept that unpleasant feelings could be discussed in this way.

The practice of asking other social workers in the social services department who speak the same language as the client, or expecting social workers from ethnic minority groups to take all the cases from that group, is also complicated. Social workers who belong to ethnic minority groups are employed to work as social workers, not as interpreters, and they may be very torn as to how to respond if asked to act as interpreter. They may be resentful that they are being used as interpreters, but they will also want to see that the person concerned receives the best possible service. This can put them in a situation of conflict – adding to the stress of their job. It may be that they are the best person for the task, but the social services department needs to have a clearly thought-out policy to which staff can refer when needed.

This is not only an issue for people whose family originally came from the 'new commonwealth'. It is equally important for people from non-English speaking groups such as Italians, Hungarians, Ukrainians, Poles, etc. When people immigrate they tend to settle with other people from the same place and so it should be possible to identify these communities locally and to ensure that good interpretation services are available.

A recent report by Patel and  on a study of twenty health care professionals who have worked with minority ethnic elders in the UK makes an interesting point. They found that 17 out of 20 respondents perceived communication to be a problem, but felt that this was not simply a language-reflected problem that could be solved by bilingual interpreters, (a suggestion that professionals emphasise). However, professionals found that some minority ethnic elders who spoke English would mix this with their mother tongue, making it difficult for the professional, the relative of the person and the translator to understand them. 'A reversion to a mother tongue among minority ethnic elders is a well-documented phenomenon and confusion often occurs in dementia' (Patel and Mirza 2000a). This is an area where much more work is needed.

A central concept of the person-centred approach is that we need to know as much as possible about the person with dementia. This task is never easy, and it is bound to be more challenging if the two people concerned come from different cultural backgrounds. However, it is of crucial importance to the making of a good assessment. The majority of social workers in this country still come from indigenous Caucasian British backgrounds. The majority are women. (The last decade has seen some improvement in the recruitment of social workers to reflect the cultural mix of this country, but the general picture still fits this description.)

## ETHNICITY

It is also very important to understand the ethnic background of the person with whom the social worker is working. An understanding of the religion, beliefs, values and customs of the ethnic group is extremely important. A person's behaviour may seem to someone from another ethnic group to be odd or difficult, and to be evidence of the progress of the dementia, but it may make perfect sense to someone who comes from the same culture. Here is a brief list of common examples of difference which cause misunderstanding:

- Body language can be very easily misinterpreted. For example, it is considered rude and disrespectful for Indian women to make direct eye contact with a person who may be perceived as possessing authority, such as a social worker. Avoiding eye contact, however, is interpreted in Caucasian British culture as being shifty, implying that the person has something to hide.

- Personal space is defined very differently in different cultures – particularly the space that is considered appropriate between men and women.

- Preferred ways of washing differ between cultures. Muslims, from wherever they originate, do not feel clean unless they wash under running water, and the same applies to many people from the Far East, such as China or Japan. However, the bath, immersing the body in water, may be very important to older Caucasian British people. Social workers will be aware that the removal of the bathing service by district nurses in recent years has caused much resentment.

- Certain kinds of clothes will mean different things to different people. People who immigrated to this country from countries which became part of the former Soviet Union may react with terror to the sight of a man in uniform, even if he is a kindly ambulance driver.

Taken out of their cultural context these reactions can very easily be misinterpreted and perceived to be examples of bizarre behaviour, which in turn is seen as further evidence of dementia.

Social workers who work with people with dementia and their families must always be aware of the possibility of misinterpretation, either of language or of culture. It is bad enough for people to battle with the dementia without having to battle with ignorance and misunderstanding as well. Value judgements are very easily based on a misunderstanding of the reason for behaviour: in spite of training in cultural awareness, health and social care professionals still make mistaken judgements based on ignorance or misunderstanding of particular cultures.

Very few social services departments can, as yet, be described as 'user friendly' to people from minority groups – which is presumably an important reason why people from these groups do not approach social services very much. One group of people who do approach social services are the families of people with dementia. Dementia is no respecter of boundaries. The disability defeats almost everybody, including members of minority ethnic groups who have a strong belief in caring for older relatives at home and whose culture still accepts the model of the extended family as the norm. It is the women in those cultures who actually do the caring, even if, as in the Asian tradition, it is the clear duty of the eldest son to look after his parents.

Most immigrants from the countries currently referred to as 'the new commonwealth' came to the United Kingdom in the 1950s and 1960s from the many Caribbean islands which make up the West Indies, and from the Indian subcontinent. If we assume that they were mostly young adults aged between twenty and thirty when they arrived, we can assume that dementia has not yet reached such significant proportions in these population groups as it has in the indigenous Caucasian population. This is because we know that most cases of Alzheimer's disease – the most common cause of dementia in Caucasian populations – occur in people aged over eighty. Therefore we can assume that dementia will only start to be a major issue for these groups during the first quarter of the twenty-first century. It would be an encouraging innovation if social services departments could learn from past mistakes and ensure that culturally appropriate services, sensitively delivered, are in place by the time when they are needed.

There is some evidence from the 'Care Needs of Ethnic Older Persons with Alzheimer's' (CNEOPSA) project that

> Black and minority ethnic organizations, in some countries, are playing an effective and important role in managing the dementia care needs of black and minority ethnic elders. These (mainstream) organizations recognise that 'BME' elders encounter two barriers when trying to attain dementia care – communication barriers (including diagnosis) which hinder them actually gaining access to services, and cultural barriers relating to inappropriate care once access has been gained. Thus, these organizations are providing information on dementia to 'BME' communities (i.e. leaflets), although audio-visual information may be more useful to these groups, to combat the communication barriers. (Patel and Mirza 2000b, p.27)

The CNEOPSA project was the first of its kind supported by the European Commission, and has now produced a video, with a booklet to accompany it. Five European countries with different minority ethnic populations took part in the project: Denmark, Finland, the Netherlands, Spain and the United Kingdom. One of the recommendations in the booklet which accompanies the training video is that: 'It is urgent that policymakers give recognition and resources to support targeted developments and research which enhance minority ethnic participation in determining appropriate dementia care'.

Following the success of the CNEOPSA project a Policy Research Institute on Ageing and Ethnicity has been established at the University of Bradford by Naina Patel and Naheed Mirza. (See Appendix Two at the end of the book.) Historically, social services departments have clung to the comforting belief that where the cultural tradition dictates that families should look after their own vulnerable and frail members, those families are still able to conform to that tradition when living in the United Kingdom. Although there are obviously examples of families who are able to do this, we know that all over the world this type of family structure is breaking down under the pressures of urbanization. However, many people from these cultural backgrounds do still retain a more cohesive family structure and a greater sense of responsibility for looking after family members. This characteristic, as well as being a feature of many Second World cultures, is apparent in some of the large European immigrant communities such as Italians and Jews, where we find a second and third generation of people who have been born in this country.

However, dementia presents all families with a major challenge, including those which are based on the extended family structure. As in all families, there is a major task of education to be undertaken in these groups about the causes, nature and progression of dementia. It is especially important to counter the belief that memory loss and confusion are part of normal ageing. But we also need to be aware that different cultures have created very different social constructs about mental health and mental illness. Some people may consider the imposition of the Western construct of dementia as a form of cultural imperialism.

If education in the Western model is felt to be appropriate and helpful to minority communities, we need to be aware that the elders of these groups may not read or write their own language, let alone English. This means that social services departments must apply lateral thinking to solving the problem of education. Money might be better spent on audiotapes than on leaflets, for example. It is useful to consider where elders from minority ethnic groups, particularly women, gather socially. A community approach, possibly through the religious structures, may be the best way forward.

The following case illustrates how the health and social care system undermined the self-esteem and apparently caused deterioration in the cognition of a man from a minority ethnic group. The experience very nearly proved fatal for him because of the failure to understand his needs and his response to the

## Case study 9

Amos Jackson was 70. He had come to the UK from Jamaica as a young man to work in a local brickworks. At home he was a lay preacher and had worked on a banana plantation. For many years he lived with Hesther, with whom he had two daughters. Amos and Hesther who was 75, lived happily together in her house. In spite of some domestic differences this arrangement worked well.

Hesther was crippled with arthritis but was able to organise the running of the home. In spite of his increasing mental impairment Amos was able to carry out Hesther's instructions. With help from social services home care, they remained independent, but Amos became more forgetful and prone to irrational outbursts of anger, and a diagnosis was made of vascular dementia. A year later he was no longer able to carry out his part of the contract. Family support was increased, but every day brought a fresh crisis. Hesther had a major stroke and was admitted to hospital. Amos would obviously not be safe alone in the house, so he went to stay with one of his daughters for a few days. She called the GP after Amos became aggressive and 'violent', and as a result he was informally admitted to the local psychiatric hospital for assessment.

From this point onwards it was downhill all the way for Amos. He had four major disadvantages. He was a man. He was a black man. He was a big black man. And he had a history of aggression. Towards the end of the three-week assessment his case was discussed in a multidisciplinary meeting. By this time he was in a sorry state, incapable of doing anything for himself. He could hardly walk and was doubly incontinent. On the basis of this evidence it was decided that he was too ill to be discharged home. He

## Case study 9 (continued)

remained in the psychiatric hospital for week after week. He lost weight and appeared to be losing language, presenting the signs of a man in the later stages of dementia. It was presumed that he had suffered another infarct, causing major cerebral damage.

Hesther's daughter, Dolores, had become the main carer for Amos. She battled for weeks to convince the hospital to reassess his case. Finally the hospital agreed to let Amos return home, provided that he received twenty-four-hour care. So, five months after his admission, he went home.

A care package for Amos and Hesther was created, with a rota of friends and family providing round-the-clock care. The social worker helped the carers to understand Amos' behaviour and worked out strategies with them to handle his behaviour. The lynchpin of the care package was Milly, who came every day with her six-year-old son, Joshua, to look after the old couple.

Within a month of returning home, Amos was back to his old self. It seemed like a miracle and he bore little resemblance to the man the social worker had seen in hospital. He was often able to hold a lucid conversation. The family took him out to church and on the bus to town. He enjoyed walking with an escort to the shops. A deeply religious man, he would spend hours listening to gospel tapes or to a portion of Scripture being read aloud to him.

Sometimes Amos thought he was in Jamaica and would insist that he had to go out into the yard to pick bananas. His suitcases remained in one of the bedrooms, packed and labelled for his return to Jamaica.

If he had stayed in the psychiatric hospital where his well-being was so severely assaulted through lack of cultural sensitivity and large amounts of antipsychotic drugs, he might well have died four years sooner than he in fact did. This is a dramatic example of the damage which can be inflicted on individuals by the health and social care system through cultural ignorance. (abbreviated version of Tibbs 1996) overwhelming strangeness of the situation in which he found himself.

## SOCIAL CLASS

This is a very real issue in this country, and one which is rarely discussed by social workers in the field of elderly care. It is uncomfortable for social workers to accept but it is nevertheless true – whether we like it or not – that there is a perception of social stigma attached to social services. For the most part, the clients of social workers are people who are on the margins of society – the physically or mentally disabled, families with internal inadequacies, children who are at risk, drug abusers, people with mental health problems, etc. The social workers who work with these people are 'tainted by association' in the public perception.

---

### Case study 10

Carol, the wife of a GP, whose father had developed vascular dementia, suddenly burst into tears as she and her mother were visiting the day centre which her father was going to attend. She and the social worker had established a good relationship and the social worker was surprised by this reaction. Through her tears Carol said, 'I just cannot bear the idea of Daddy climbing into one of those bright green social services buses. It is so degrading. People like us don't use social services. We are used to offering help to other people when they need it – not receiving it from social workers.'

This family developed an excellent relationship with the social worker, the day centre and the residential home during the five-year course of Carol's father's illness. He had been the headmaster of a private school, but never had any problems with prejudice against social services – although many people do have problems in trying to make sense of an environment which is totally unfamiliar.

---

It comes as a shock to middle-class families, therefore, when they have to turn to social services for help when their relative develops dementia. They have no problem approaching the medical profession. Everyone has a doctor. But when they discover that social services is the gatekeeper of the help which they so desperately need, this knowledge may be unwelcome. Middle-class people also tend to be more able to stand up for their rights and the rights of those for whom they are acting as advocates. They want to know, and feel they have a right to know, all the details of the care package and the reasons why particular decisions were made. And they are confident enough to request more information about decisions. They may even challenge those decisions. For this reason they are very easily perceived as troublemakers. The social services system is not always geared to working with people like this. For the most part its clients are inarticulate and powerless, even in their anger and frustration, because they cannot express their feelings clearly.

In the case of the oldest people in our communities, many are still pitifully grateful for the little which is offered to them. So social workers, as well as other community health workers, become defensive and even feel hostile when faced with people who are empowered.

Dementia, as we know, can strike anybody – right across the social spectrum. This explains why social workers in this field will have a disproportionately high percentage of cases where the family is articulate, empowered in the sense that they know how to complain. They will do so, and will readily challenge the decisions made by professionals. If we are going to use a person-centred approach (including person-centred assessments) then this factor has to be taken into account. Social class defines people just as much as gender, ethnicity, religion or sexual orientation.

Because of the prevalence of dementia, social workers working with this client group are likely to have several families on their caseload who have never dreamed, prior to this crisis in their lives, of approaching social services for help. At this point they will have to do so. In order to receive the practical help (such as day care, residential respite care, advice on benefits and legal and financial issues) which they need, they will have to make themselves known to social services. They will have to be referred, a case file will be generated and they will acquire a social services PIN number – the bureaucratic system will take hold of them. Social workers need to be aware that this in itself can be difficult for many people, because it is so alien to them. Many people are still unclear about the difference between social services and the Benefits Agency, causing further misunderstandings initially.

It is always difficult to judge a culture from within. Most social workers are unaware that the social services departments they work in have a culture of their own. It is to a great extent still a closed world, with its own language and jargon and procedures often so complex and idiosyncratic that they are incomprehensible to those outside. People working within the culture spend most of their working lives talking to other people who share the same history and experience. They often do not realize how difficult it is for people outside to comprehend the procedures – let alone the reasons for them. Social workers need to be aware of this in their practice, instead of assuming that they are a totally neutral, professional person going into the situation, free of prejudice and never making value-judgements. Social workers, like their colleagues in the health care professions, are trained to be all these things, but the culture in which they work often has a profound effect upon them – although this is rarely examined in any critical way. People who do not conform to the social services client stereotype may often be labelled 'difficult'.

# AGE
## Early onset dementia

Because the incidence of dementia rises sharply from the age of 65, the issue of dementia is of most significance to social workers in teams working with older people, which is why the emphasis of this book is directed towards work with this age group. However, social workers should be aware that there are 17,000 people under the age of 65 with dementia in the UK at present (Alzheimer's Society Information Section, 2000).

A person's age will affect their experience and response to dementia in the same way as ethnicity and social class, so younger people have unique circumstances which need unique services. Yet in many places there are no age-specific services available. People have to be fitted into amenities, such as day centres and respite care, which have been developed to meet the needs of the very elderly population. Activities such as reminiscence about the 1930s and 1940s, gentle physical activities such as carpet bowls and skittles, community singing of war-time songs, or watching videos of the royal family are not likely to hold much significance for active people with early onset dementia.

It is very important that age sensitive services are provided in every area – even if there are not many younger people with dementia who need them. It is no longer acceptable to offer them and their families the existing services, which cannot meet their needs, on the grounds that the local authority or health authority cannot afford anything else.

As differential diagnosis becomes more common we are able to identify the different causes of dementia, and people with early onset dementia are much more likely to be in a research programme than older people. Certain conditions are now identified much more specifically than was previously the case. For example, Picks disease and frontal lobe dementia are now thought to be responsible for 5 per cent of the total cases of dementia, whereas in the past they would probably have been labelled as Alzheimer's disease. Many of these people would fall into the group we refer to as early onset dementia. Sporadic Alzheimer's disease is still thought to account for 55 per cent of cases in people of all ages (Alzheimer's Society Information Section 2000). Hereditary Alzheimer's disease is extremely rare, as is new variant CJD. The figures for AIDS-related dementia and Huntington's chorea are also small. A group of people who are at increased risk of developing Alzheimer's disease are those with Down syndrome: Alzheimer's disease is relatively common in people with Down syndrome over the age of forty.

Younger people are more likely to be taking one of the drugs for symptomatic treatment of Alzheimer's disease, such as Aricept and Exelon. This is the group of people who are able to tell us what it is like to have dementia, and their voice is beginning to be heard. They need early diagnosis and services within easy reach which are designed to meet their needs. Their carers also have needs for information and support, which differ somewhat from those of older people. The Alzheimer's Society has a small group of younger people in the early stages of dementia, with whom they are able to consult about the services they need, and who can suggest the type of support they want. This means that for the first time we are really hearing from individuals who can describe their own needs. This has happened through the Society's "Younger Person Project" a new project which has a dedicated project worker. There are now a few specialized units for younger people with dementia in different parts of the country.

The challenge of caring for a younger person with dementia can be very great. The person may be working when the condition develops, and so financial hardship is an added factor for their family. Carers of these people are often very angry as well as bewildered. In some types of dementia there is the additional burden of fear that the person's children may inherit the condition. These families need very intensive support. In some areas the specialist services which younger people need have been established, and they are becoming more visible as a group, and better served than was the case five years ago.

## SEXUAL ORIENTATION

The statutory health and social care system tends to assume that all couples are heterosexual and probably married. We, as a society, are now recognizing that marriage is no longer the norm, and we are also increasingly prepared to acknowledge the existence of long-term same-sex partnerships. People with dementia are simply part of the whole population, and so we will come across same-sex couples where one partner develops dementia.

There are particular problems for these people.

The lack of any kind of investigation into the experiences of lesbians and gay men affected by dementia hampers dementia care professionals in their understanding and ability to respond appropriately to this community. As indeed does the paucity of research into the experiences of older gays and lesbians generally. (Ward 2000, p.25)

When today's oldest generation were young, homosexuality was illegal and so they may have had a lifetime of secrecy about their sexual orientation. Their social class, occupation and the place where they live will have affected this, but people of their generation were not able to live openly in same-sex relationships, as it is possible to do now. In order to be recognized as the life-long partner of a person with dementia, homosexual carers may have to 'come out' to the person's family for the first time. This may be quite straightforward but, conversely, may have catastrophic effects on all concerned. It is an area of potential conflict, of which the social worker should be aware.

There is now a national helpline for homosexual and lesbian carers. The number can be obtained from the Alzheimer's Society. (See Appendix Two at the end of this book.)

Sensitive awareness and a capacity for empathy are attributes which are particularly important for the dementia-specific social worker, especially when working with members of minority groups.

## SUMMARY

- A person's language, ethnic background, social class, age and sexual orientation will shape their experience of and response to dementia. Social workers need to be fully aware of the ways in which these influences can impact on the way individuals respond to the services which are available.

- There is clearly a need to ensure that services are available which are culturally sensitive to the needs of clients from minority groups.

- Social workers need to think laterally in order to ensure that minority needs are met, and mainstream resources such as day centres and luncheon clubs for elders from specific minority ethnic groups may, for example, be the most appropriate way to offer support. If this is the case, the people running such centres will need additional training on the special needs of people with dementia.

# CHAPTER SEVEN

# The Road Ahead – Directions for the Future

## INTRODUCTION

In this final chapter we shall look at some trends in government policy which are emerging in recognition of the fact that the delivery of social care needs modernization. This will clearly affect the practice of social work in future.

This seems, therefore, an appropriate time to look at ways in which social work for people with dementia and their carers might be restructured in order to deliver a better service. Finally, I propose a model for a dementia-specific social work service to meet the needs of this group of people for effective, focused assessment and intervention and ongoing, specialist support which can be sustained over a long period of time.

## FURTHER REFORM OF THE DELIVERY OF SOCIAL CARE IS PLANNED

Since 1997 the new administration had begun to reform the NHS and the social care system. Several important policies and initiatives have been launched. Some of these recent government documents are likely to have profound implications for the delivery of social care. I propose to examine four of these documents that are particluarly relevant to social work in this field: Modernising Social Services (Department of Health

1998), *With Respect to Old Age* (Sutherland 1999), Reform of the Mental Health Act (Department of Health 1997) and Making Decisions (Lord Chancellor's Office 1999). It is useful to examine the implications of these for social work with dementia.

## The government White Paper 'Modernising Social Services' (1998)

Social workers may or may not greet with delight the news that further reform of their profession is on its way. However, some of the facts given in the White Paper make interesting reading and are clearly significant for our field. The document clearly reflects the view that social services, while being an essential part of a caring society, are not adequately fulfilling their role.

In the introduction to the White Paper a clear and convincing case is made for the reform of social services, pointing to the fact that

> factors such as demographic changes, and changes in the patterns of family life are likely to mean that the need for social services will increase in the coming years. With recent increases in health care, more people, including those with profound disabilities, are able to live longer, and they rely on effective social services to achieve more fulfilling lives. (Department of Health 1998, p.4)

The document makes the point that 'Social services does not just support a small number of "social casualties" but is an important part of the fabric of a caring society' (p.5). This reflects the reality of social work with dementia where, as we have seen, all sections of society are affected and even the extended family structure is often unable to handle the situation without outside help. Families caring for a person with dementia can obviously not be classed as 'social casualties'.

Many people are now employed in the field of social care

The document goes on to point out that

> social care has been one of the fastest growing employment sectors in recent years and the workforce now numbers around one million ... two thirds of them in the independent sector (*mainly working with old people in residential homes, about 40% of whom show evidence of dementia* [my italics]) ... 80% of this large workforce which works directly with very vulnerable people have no qualifications or training ... only 40,000 or so are professionally qualified social workers. (p.84)

The White Paper stresses that, in spite of the fact that social care is one of the fastest growing employment sectors, this workforce is inadequately praised or recompensed for its role.

## Eligibility criteria

The issue of eligibility criteria is addressed in the document. Local authorities were instructed to provide clear criteria about who is eligible for their services, under the NHS and Community Care act 1990. In the years since 1993 when the community care section was implemented local authorities, responding to inadequate financial resources, have increasingly been using the eligibility criteria as a means of rationing services. Local authorities have been allowed to frame their own eligibility criteria, which has created a very unequal service in different parts of the country. The White Paper states that

> eligibility criteria are getting ever tighter and excluding more and more people who would benefit from help but who do not come into the most dependent categories. Decisions about care can still be service driven and concentrate on doing things for people according to what is available rather than tailoring services to the needs of individuals and encouraging those who are helped to do what they can for themselves. (p.13)

This is clearly an area where reform may be expected.

## The contribution of carers

In section 2.10 the report makes the point that

> the care system does not adequately recognise the enormous
> contribution that informal carers make to maintaining the
> independence of people with care needs. Carers are the most
> important providers of social care: according to the 1995
> General Household Survey of Great Britain, they number 5.7
> million, with 1.7 million of them providing care for 20 hours
> or more each week. (p.15)

## General Social Care Council

The Government also intends to create a new General Social
Care Council (GSCC – see Chapter 5 of the White Paper), which
will replace the Central Council for Education and Training in
Social Work (CCETSW) in regulating the training of social
workers, will set conduct and practice standards, and register
those working in the most sensitive areas.

It proposes that the GSCC will have a registration function.
'Soon after its establishment the GSCC will open a register of
people who have obtained a professional social work qualification...' It intends to provide for periodic re-registration to
be introduced when the Secretary of State considers it appropriate because it is common in other professions for continued
registration to be linked to continuing professional education
and development.

## Lack of consistency of service

The White Paper identified a major problem caused by lack of
consistency among local authorities. In section 2.26 it states

> The ways in which needs are assessed and the routes through
> which people gain access to services, can vary from authority

to authority, or even within a single authority. The result is (section 2.27) that someone with long-term care needs might receive high level care in their own homes from social services and the NHS in one place, whereas in another they might have to go into residential or nursing-home care. (p.23)

## With Respect to Old Age

As the placing of people with dementia in long-term care homes forms such a large part of the social work task today, together with the financial assessments which are central to the process, this report of the Royal Commission into the Funding of Long-Term Care is of considerable interest to social workers in the field.

The Royal Commission into the Funding of Long-Term Care was appointed shortly after the 1997 General Election and published its report in March 1999 (Sutherland 1999). The obvious unfairness and general unpopularity of the system of funding which had developed during the 1980s had become a political issue. The resource implications for the government would be enormous if the system were significantly changed, because of the number of people involved. We should be aware that many of these people have dementia. Here is a clear example of the fact that the government has to find new solutions, both for long-standing problems and for new problems now facing us.

The report is entitled *With Respect to Old Age*. Social workers will find it encouraging that the Royal Commission made clear that it found the present system seriously deficient in several ways.

The current system is particularly characterised by complexity and unfairness in the way it operates. It has grown up piecemeal and apparently haphazardly over the years. It contains a number of providers and funders of care, each of whom has different management or financial interests which may work against the interests of the individual client. (Chapter 4, p.2)

This is an important issue, which has to be resolved. It is rendered more acute by the fact that our population is ageing significantly. Currently there is an unusually high percentage of very old people in the population. These are the people born between 1915 and 1925 – the 'babyboomers' of World War I – who are now over 85. Because of the health needs associated with extreme old age, this large group is placing a great strain on the health and social care systems.

*With Respect to Old Age* refers in section 4.7 to the startling fact that

the number of NHS long-stay beds has reduced by 38% since 1983 (a loss of 21,300 beds), and the number of private nursing home places has increased by 900% (an increase of 141,000 beds). (Chapter 4, p.4)

In section 4.8 the report states that

Only 8% of these additional private nursing home places are paid for by health authorities and health boards. The rest are paid for by individuals, or by local authorities. The total saving to the NHS over this period, also taking into account the cheaper nursing home beds funded by the NHS as a substitute for long-stay hospital beds, was considerable. It is difficult to tell but there remains a lingering suspicion that, in order to concentrate its resources on acute care, the NHS has been increasingly reluctant to provide long term care for older people. (Chapter 4, p.4)

The report recommends that the Government should conduct a scrutiny of the shift in resources supporting long-term care since the early 1980s, and should consider whether there should be a transfer of resources between the NHS and social services budgets, given changes in relative responsibilities. (Recommendation 4.2) (Chapter 4, p.2)

Care homes standards for dementia care

An encouraging development in the field of residential care is the proposed publication, for the first time, of dementia-specific standards. These standards are the result of a collaboration between the Alzheimer's Society and the Royal College of Nursing. Published in January 2001 under the title of 'Quality dementia care in care homes – person centred standards.'

## 'Reform of the Mental Health Act'

As we have seen in Chapter Three, the Mental Health Act has serious limitations as a tool to protect the interests of people with dementia. Social workers in the field are aware that reform is long overdue, and the fact that reform is proposed must be welcome.

Until quite recently, custom and practice dictated that people with dementia were often moved from their own homes without their consent and without the protection of the law. There was a belief among social workers, including approved social workers, that using the Act to 'section' a 'little old lady' was unduly harsh and punitive. Guardianship (Section 7 of the Act), as we saw (p.50), has proved to be of limited use, although it was intended to meet the needs of mentally impaired adults, including people with dementia.

The government is currently in the process of reforming the Mental Health Act and has published a consultation paper on the subject, Reform of the Mental Health Act (Lord Chancellor's Department, 1999). The document points out that

> the last review of mental health legislation took place in the 1950s, which led to the establishment of a framework that has been in place for nearly 40 years. During that time there have been major changes because of the development of new drugs, a growing understanding of the role of other therapeutic approaches, and recognition of the important

part that social care plays in treatment and support of people with a mental disorder. (Chapter 2, p.1)

Chapter 11 of the consultation proposals deals with safeguards for people with long-term mental incapacity. It is recognized that detention under the Mental Health Act is often inappropriate. But 'these people do need statutory safeguards to ensure that care and treatment for mental disorder, particularly when restrictions of liberty are concerned, is in their best interests' (Chapter 11, p.1).

## 'Making Decisions' Government Report 1999

This is an area of law, and consequently social work practice, which is so complex that no government has yet managed to find an acceptable balance between the two opposing duties. These are the state's duty to protect the individual freedoms of everyone, including adults who lack mental capacity, and the duty to protect such people from harm. Reform in this area, as in the Mental Health Act, will be very welcome to social workers who are struggling with these issues on a day-to-day basis.

The Mental Health Act 1983, flawed as it is, provides the only form of protection we have for the 'person' of an individual who lacks mental capacity. There is a far more comprehensive structure to protect the property and finances of such people, with the powers currently held by the Court of Protection. This state of affairs may reflect the relative importance which we as a society attach to civil liberties and to property.

The report sets out proposals to 'provide a clear, consistent framework – giving certainty and protection to people who need to make decisions for those unable to do so'. A new statutory test of capacity will clarify the law. It will include a statutory presumption against 'lack of capacity' and protect the incapacitated by stating that all practicable steps must be taken to enable them to communicate their own decisions.

In our field this seems to mean that professionals and carers who are planning to act against the stated wishes of a person with dementia will have to demonstrate to the court that the person with dementia is in practice mentally incapacitated. At present it is still possible to presume that the person lacks mental capacity because a diagnosis of dementia has been made. There will be a legal safeguard for carers and professionals, and protection for those they look after, in all day-to-day decisions that must be taken. Two new proposals are:

1. The creation of a new Continuing Power of Attorney which will allow people to nominate trusted friends to make decisions on their behalf on matters of health, welfare and finance if they become mentally incapable at some future date. This will replace the existing Enduring Power of Attorney.

2. The creation of a new Court of Protection to deal with all areas of decision-making in cases of adult mental incapacity. The new Court will sit in the regions instead of only in London, as is the case at present.

The policy statement was issued following the publication of the Law Commission's report entitled *Who Decides?* (Lord Chancellor's Office 1997b) which had considered the subject from 1990 to 1995, consulting very thoroughly with all interested parties.

The government is clearly taking a long, hard look at social work with clients of all ages. This must include people with dementia. It seems to be an appropriate time, therefore, to look at ways in which the service can be improved.

## The Forget Me Not Report (2000)

A report published in January 2000 by the Audit Commission examined mental health services for older people in twelve health authorities. It provides evidence-based research on the state of mental health services for older people as they were in 1999/2000 and will confirm what most social workers in the field know from their own experience.

Not surprisingly it highlights, as other reports have done, the fact that at present the number of very old people (people over 80) is the fastest growing group in the population. One-quarter of that population develops dementia. One-third of the people over 80 with dementia need twenty-four-hour supervision and/or care.

The report states that

> the cost of caring has been estimated at £6.1 billion (at 1998/9 prices) for older people with dementia. Almost one-half of these costs fall to unpaid family carers, who may also be old or have mental health problems of some kind themselves. (Audit Commission 2000, p.2)

The carers of these people are in urgent need of help. Half of the carers surveyed said that the GP had not told them what the problem was or how it was likely to affect them. Only four of the twelve areas studied had readily available written information for carers. Less than half of the GPs consulted felt that they had sufficient training to diagnose and manage dementia. Less than half the GPs were currently using a standard test to measure cognitive impairment. Specialist help to residential and nursing homes was found to be patchy, with only four of the twelve areas providing specialist teams to support the staff of residential and nursing homes. Only four of the twelve areas have joint commissioning arrangements between health and social services in place.

It is encouraging to see that the report advocates dementia care mapping (DCM) for use in long-term care homes, stating that

> Dementia Care mapping (DCM) for monitoring the environment experienced by users, can make a great deal of

difference. Learning to undertake DCM and getting feedback from it can greatly enhance the awareness and understanding of staff and improve the care they provide. Visits from specialists to monitor the quality of care and support staff can be beneficial for both users and staff. (See Bradford Dementia Group with Kitwood, T.) (p.2)

The report concluded that people who would otherwise need residential care could live at home if provided with flexible home-based care provided by joint health and social services teams. They found evidence that people with dementia can regain living skills.

It is my belief that we need to re-examine the question of where, within the traditional client groupings, people with dementia are placed. We should consider whether they should be made into a specific client group.

I believe that the short-term model of working does not best serve people with dementia and their carers. They need ongoing assessment and support in the same way as do people with physical and learning disabilities.

## A DIFFERENT APPROACH IS NEEDED

It seems to me that the way social work for people with dementia is currently structured fails to meet the needs of those it is intended to serve. The care management model works well for generic care of older people and is well suited to the large volume and high turnover of these cases. Most of these people will only need social work intervention for short periods of time while they are affected by a temporary disability or period of emotional distress.

People with dementia have needs which are quite different. As we saw in Chapter Two, they are travellers on a journey which may last for many years. What they and their carers need above all is the knowledge that expert help and good support services exist and can be rapidly reached when needed. This means that the current practice of 'closing cases' after an initial assessment and creation of a care package does not meet the needs of clients. In fact, it seems to exacerbate their feelings of frustration and insecurity.

## We need a disability model for people with dementia

We are moving away from the concept and language of disease and suffering in relation to dementia. A disability model has much to recommend it as an alternative. If a person has a physical or learning disability they are likely to receive ongoing social-work support, but a person with dementia over sixty-five will not receive the same service unless s/he is fortunate enough to live in an area with a specialist team which uses this model.

People with dementia should be regarded as disabled, rather than as suffering from a disease. Alzheimer's disease can last up to twenty years. Surely a disability model would be more appropriate to the care needs of such people and their families? People live with a disability, and disabled people have rights. This may seem like a mere play on words, but it is an important issue which needs addressing. The distinction is a narrow one, but it is very significant. The universal adoption of the term 'Alzheimer's disease' to describe dementia has in some sense been counterproductive. The social construct of dementia which has become the standard paradigm is the medical model, which is described by Kitwood in the following way:

> Essentially the paradigm frames the problems surrounding dementia in a technical way, as an electronics expert might with a computer whose hardware is faulty, or a mechanic with a car that has broken down. (Kitwood 1997, p.37).

This view sees the brain almost as a reality which exists in a vacuum. It takes no account of the person in whose body that brain exists. The standard paradigm has been accepted so widely because, for most of its history up until the past five years, the medical profession has been unable to offer any means of either affecting the course of the dementia or of treating the symptoms arising from it. The conclusion drawn from these facts was that there was nothing at all that anyone could do to help. But 'The standard paradigm ... does not tell us the truth about dementia. "Alzheimer's: no cure, no help, no hope" is a false proposition; the "death that leaves the body behind" is a misleading image' (Kitwood 1997, p.37).

On the other hand, the great advantage of the general acceptance of the term 'Alzheimer's disease' is that it has passed into popular usage, and public awareness of the condition has grown enormously. From public awareness grows pressure for better services, empowerment of people with dementia and those who care for them, and greater allocation of public funds. It is difficult to create the right balance between these two approaches.

## People with dementia are a distinct client group

They need social workers who have specialist training

We have seen throughout this book that strategies which constitute good practice for work with older people who are not mentally impaired do not work well for those with dementia. Specialist social-work skills are needed.

It seems clear to me from experience that bolting social work with people with dementia onto social work with older people is not an effective working model. As we have seen, 40 per cent of the caseloads of many area social-work teams for the elderly represent people with dementia and, in order to work with them appropriately, specialist training is needed. In a study by Levin and Webb (1997) one of the areas of training need clearly identified by social workers themselves was 'in issues related to dementia and mental health work with older people' (p.20).

A more satisfactory solution for people with dementia, for those who care for them, and for those who work with them in a professional capacity, would be to make them into a distinct client group. This means creating a specialism within the care of older people and providing additional ongoing support and training for staff.

## The arbitrary division of services on the basis of chronological age is not always the best solution for people with dementia

As we saw in Chapter Six, people with early onset dementia have different needs to the majority of people with dementia, who are aged over 75. Whether or not to divide people on the basis of age is a difficult decision.

There is an implicit ageism in the assumption that people over 65 are 'elderly' and need a particular type of service, and that those under 65 have different needs. Many people who are over 65 enjoy good health and are extremely active. As social workers who work with older people know, the vast majority of their cases are of people aged 75 and over.

The division of adult clients into age-groups means that people with early onset dementia, because they are younger, may be placed under the care of social workers whose cases are not usually people with dementia. The situation is not simple. One reason for placing these clients within physical disability teams is because it means that they may have access to a larger budget, because there are so few clients in this age-group compared to the over-75 age range. Also, it is more likely that the disability model will be applied to the work done with them. However, it is to their disadvantage that social workers for people who develop early onset dementia may find themselves cut off from the existing body of dementia expertise. The person who holds their case is likely to have very few cases of people with dementia on his/her caseload, and little opportunity to build up experience and develop the specialist skills needed for this work.

## Flexibility is very important

It is in the nature of dementia, and the response of others to it, that situations change with great rapidity. Social workers have to be prepared to change care plans with great frequency.

If the practice issues which we examined in Chapter Four are addressed, people with dementia and their carers will enjoy a much better quality of life, and the situation will not collapse into a crisis as is often the case at present. There are usually long periods of time between crisis points when the case can be transferred to the 'non-active' list. Equally, there are periods when something seems to change every week. Social workers in this field have to accept the fact that a care plan which has been developed using much time and thought may have to be changed in some detail the following week, and abandoned altogether the week after. This reflects how the needs of the person change and, perhaps more significantly, how carers respond to the demands which are placed upon them.

## Disseminating good practice

Nobody wants to be in the business of reinventing wheels. We need to learn from good practice in different parts of the country so that what we have learned can be transmitted easily from one place to another. There have been isolated examples of good practice in dementia care for many years now, but for some reason they do not seem to have entered the mainstream. Mainstream practice still remains traditional – over-bureaucratic and lacking the multidisciplinary approach which is clearly needed.

# WE NEED A NEW MODEL FOR A COMMUNITY SERVICE FOR PEOPLE WITH DEMENTIA
## A one-stop shop with a single point of entry

We know, from talking to carers for many years, that they find it very difficult to pick their way through the labyrinth of bureaucracy which confronts them when dementia is diagnosed. There are just no signposts to show them the way. We know that many GPs do not divulge the diagnosis. Others give a diagnosis but do not explain what it means. They do not refer their patients on at all for social support, and many carers have a long period of time in which they would like help but do not know what help they need or what is available. (The Forget Me Not (2000) report has provided evidence for this.)

If there is a specialist team geographically separate from the area office and easily accessible to them, carers can be appropriately supported. Once they have told their story and been entered in the system, they do not want to have to keep repeating it to other people. This is one of the things which carers tell us they find particularly difficult to cope with.

Carers need to have confidence that social workers know what they are doing, and to be able to trust them.

## A multidisciplinary team

Almost all people with dementia have health needs as well as social care needs. The great chasm between the two halves of the statutory system (health and social services) does not help the person with dementia and their carer at all. There is a great need for what is referred to in government documents as 'joined-up' working in order to provide a 'seamless service'. The rhetoric is appealing but the goal still proves elusive.

Community psychiatric nurses are doing a very similar job to social workers in many areas and there may be duplication of time and effort. In the past a family where a member has dementia may have been subjected to the visits of several different professionals, all doing their own separate assessments. This is confusing and sometimes distressing for the person and their carer. It has also led to some clients receiving help from several quarters and others receiving none. We therefore must have a multidisciplinary approach. The exact form that takes will differ from place to place depending on the local history and geography.

## Cases should be kept 'open'

It is clear that what carers need is to know that somebody is there who is 'their' contact person, to whom they can turn when they need help. They need to have a name and a phone number which they can ring when the going gets rough along the journey through the care system. We know that we may be talking about a period of several years.

The care management model of allocating cases, making an initial assessment, setting up the care package and then closing the case (apart from reviews) works well for short-term interventions with physically frail older people. But it is not appropriate for this client group. We have examined the reasons why this is so.

## People need ongoing support

In order to keep a case open, ongoing support is needed. This role is already being developed in restricted areas within the voluntary sector, with the Admiral Nurse Scheme and some branches of the Alzheimer's Society. It may be possible to look at combinations of workers who support a family on a long-term basis. The support role does not need to be performed by a qualified social worker whose time is expensive. Partnerships with the voluntary sector may be the best way forward. It is often argued that such an approach is too costly. However, experience would seem to suggest that extra money spent at this end of the journey would be saved at the other end because the person is likely to be supported much longer by the family or friends. It is not easy to prove or disprove this perception, which is derived from personal experience. Even the Royal Commission on Long Term Care (Sutherland 1999) states that

> No-one really knows just how much public or private money goes to support older people in long-term care. Despite our best efforts in the time available, we have been unable to shed definitive light on this matter. (p.3)

In the same way, we cannot be certain how many people go into care before they need to, because the carer cannot continue.

The question of whether a person with dementia is always best cared for at home for as long as the carer feels able to do so, is also complex, and further research into this question is needed.

## Primary dementia care teams need psychologists

Psychologists have played and continue to play a significant role in the development of the new culture of dementia care. Psycho-therapy with people in the early stages of dementia, as well as with carers, is now being carried out successfully. Psychologists can also offer alternative strategies to medication in working with behaviour, which is sometimes so hard for carers (paid and unpaid) to live with. An increasing number of professionals in the field are realizing that using psychotropic medication to suppress symptoms of agitation and aggression is not a long-term solution (Hopker 1999). The pain and distress felt by the person has to go somewhere, and will appear in the form of physical symptoms or different behavioural reactions.

## The importance of gathering qualitative information

The present system of assessment, and the paperwork that it has generated, is quantitative and does not readily allow for an in-depth, ongoing process to be recorded. The drive is for social workers to fill in forms for statisticians to analyse, so that the 'number-crunching' required by the process of monitoring and evaluation can continue. Unfortunately, this can work against good practice. Computerization means that it is now relatively easy to obtain quantitative information, and this has come to be perceived as being essential and of intrinsic worth.

It is much more difficult to obtain qualitative information and so, although lip service is paid to 'quality assurance', much less attention and value is, in reality, attached to it. This is as true in the field of dementia care as in any other client group. But it is qualitative information that we need at the moment.

We need to know what works and what does not work for users of services and their carers, in order to develop a model of best practice. We need to find a way to record the opinions of people with dementia and those who care for them about the services they receive

## CONCLUSION

In conclusion let us return to the image that we started with in Chapter Two – the journey through the social care system, which is made by the person with dementia and their carers. These people follow a track which is hard to detect initially, but which turns into a clear pathway as the cognitive decline becomes more marked. They need to know where they are going and what they are likely to encounter on the way. The places where problems can be predicted should be clearly marked, and help should be available at those points. The travellers should be able to contact help all the way along the route, however long the journey lasts. Guides who are well trained and well equipped should be available, and if there is an emergency the travellers should know where and how to summon the emergency services. Social workers and CPNs should be as reliable and as swift in offering help in emergencies as the paramedics and fire officers who come in response to a road traffic accident or fire. People have a right to expect that this should be so.

If social workers are the guides on this pathway, they will need to develop a high level of knowledge and expertise in their chosen specialism. Because people with dementia and their carers have unique needs, situations arise which are both complex and challenging. Often, there are no easy solutions. We are not pretending that this is an easy area in which to work.

It is no accident that the part of social work with older people in which person centred care has developed is the field of dementia care. This is because practice was so bad in the old culture of dementia care, when people were cared for in the old psychiatric institutions. A reaction against it was generated. But we need to be aware that the asylum still casts a long shadow, and much current care practice still takes place within that shadow, even though most of the asylums are now closed. It is the mental attitudes associated with them, that are still deeply rooted in our culture.

Imaginative and creative ways of working with people with dementia are being developed in this and other countries – the use of poetry to communicate (Killick 1997), the use of play and the creative arts, alternative therapies, a growing interest in spirituality and dementia (Shamy 1997) and the use of reminiscence (Schweitzer 1998). All these are examples of pioneering work in this field.

Best practice developed in the field of dementia care should enter the field of generic care for older people and for people with other disabilities, whose needs may be different in degree but not in essence from those who are mentally impaired. Social work with people with dementia, therefore, places practitioners at the cutting edge of best practice in the field of care for older people. The days when it was known as 'the Cinderella service' have long gone.

The challenge which faces us is very great, but so is the opportunity to develop new ideas and strategies as we move forward together into an exciting period of change in social and health care services.

# Financial and Legal Expertise

## INTRODUCTION

It is of vital importance that social workers working with people with dementia are competent in financial and legal matters. In a situation where the main client is a person who, in all probability, is no longer able to take responsibility for making their own financial decisions because of their impaired cognitive ability, it is very important that the interests of all are safeguarded.

## A SHORT GUIDE FOR MANAGING THE FINANCIAL AFFAIRS OF A PERSON WITH DEMENTIA

I have compiled this guide from my own experience to assist social workers in this task.

### The nomination of an appointee

Such a person is authorized by the Benefits Agency to receive and administer benefits on behalf of another person. Appointeeship is useful in situations where the only income is from benefits. It cannot be used to conduct any other financial transactions or to gain access to capital assets. Contact has to be made with the local office of the Benefits Agency so that a nominated person can be made appointee in order to cash those benefits.

## The making of an Enduring Power of Attorney

For this to be made, the person who is making it has to be aware of what they are doing and consent to it. Therefore this step should be taken as soon as possible after the diagnosis has been made. The donor of the power of attorney has to convince a solicitor that they possess the mental capacity to do so. People normally give their Power of Attorney to a relative, partner or close friend whom they trust, who becomes the 'Attorney'.

The Enduring Power of Attorney came into existence in 1986. It allows a person to decide whom they would want to administer their financial affairs in the event of loss of mental capacity and – unlike the ordinary Power of Attorney – does not lapse when the person loses such mental capacity.

## When the person is assessed medically as no longer possessing mental capacity the Enduring Power of Attorney is registered with the Court of Protection

The 'Attorney' then no longer needs the consent of the person with dementia to act on their behalf. These powers cover all financial decisions up to and including the sale of property. The Court of Protection is an office of the Supreme Court and is currently still based in London. The Protection Division of the Public Trust Office deals with the day-to-day administration of cases under the jurisdiction of the Court, which is an Executive Agency within the Lord Chancellor's Department.

## If nobody has addressed the issue of the management of the financial affairs until the person with dementia has lost mental capacity then an application has to be made to place them under the Court of Protection

Someone, usually a relative, is named as Receiver and administers their finances in their name. There are certain circumstances in which it is advisable to place the person under the protection of the court:

- If there is conflict within a family which seems likely to impact on the finances, it is good practice for the social worker to advise or even approach a solicitor to act on behalf of the person. Social services departments would not usually agree to act as Receivers because of the resource implications.

- If a person is living alone, with no relatives involved in their care, and possesses significant financial assets, such as a house, it is always advisable to approach a solicitor to act on their behalf.

## Many social workers are unaware of the Short Procedure Order of the Court of Protection

This can be used effectively to help a person who is living on benefits, with minimal resources, and on whose behalf a legal transaction, such as the termination of a tenancy, has to be conducted. As in all branches of the law, some solicitors have considerable expertise in this field while others are relatively ignorant. It is not safe to assume that all solicitors will have much experience in this area of the law. Social workers should take active steps to discover which solicitors in their locality specialize in this area of the law. With the ageing population, there are now more of them to be found than there were in the past. (LawNet is an organization of lawyers which works in association with the Alzheimer's Society. They will provide a list of solicitors in the area who are registered with them. See Appendix Two at the end of this book)

## The existence of a will

It is surprising how many relatives of people with dementia assume that, because a will was made when the person was mentally capable, disposing of their assets, the matter needs no further attention. It is sometimes necessary to point out the obvious basic fact that a will only takes effect when a person has died. Decisions about finance still have to be made during the person's lifetime.

Various organizations (e.g. Age Concern, the Alzheimer's Society) produce leaflets and fact-sheets explaining financial and legal matters and providing useful contact numbers for further information and advice. It is good practice for social workers to carry these and leave them for carers to read and refer to after the social worker has left.

The impact of dementia on other family members cannot be underestimated. Feelings of distress and denial undermine people's ability to take in information and to make rational decisions. At highly stressful points in the process, such as the time when permanent residence in long-term care is necessary, these difficulties are likely to be intensified. This is why it is so important for social workers to think ahead and to encourage their clients to tackle these issues early on. It may need many discussions, covering the same ground more than once, before carers are able to bring themselves to take action which to those outside the family seems the obvious and sensible thing to do.

# Some Useful Contacts for Social Workers

### Age Concern England
Astral House
1268 London Road
London SW16 4ER
Tel: 020 8679 8000
email: ace@ace.org.uk
http://www.ace.org.uk

### Age Concern Scotland
113 Rose Street
Edinburgh EH2 3DT
Tel: 0131 220 3345
email: enquiries@acs.freeserve.co.uk

### Age Exchange Theatre Trust
The Reminiscence Centre
11 Blackheath Village
London SE3 9LA
Tel: 020 8318 9105
email: age-exchange@lewisham.gov.uk

### The Alzheimer's Society (England, Wales and Northern Ireland)
Gordon House
10 Greencoat Place
London SW1P 1PH
Tel: 020 7306 0606
email: info@alzheimers.org.uk (on letterheads)
http:// www.alzheimers.org.uk

### Alzheimer Scotland – Action on Dementia
22 Drumsheugh Gardens
Edinburgh EH3 7RN
Tel: 0131 243 1453
email: Alzheimer@alzscot.org
http://www.alzscot.org

## Bradford Dementia Group
School of Health Studies
University of Bradford
West Yorks BD7 1DP
Tel: 01274 233996
email: m.downs@bradford.ac.uk
http://www.brad.ac.uk/acad/health/dementia.htm

## C.A.N.D.I.D
(Counselling and Diagnosis in Dementia)
National Hospital for Neurology and Neurosurgery
Queen Square
London WC1N 3BG
Tel: 020 7829 8772
email: enquiries@dementia.ion.ucl.ac.uk
http://www.dementia.ion.ucl

## Carers National Association
20–25 Glasshouse Yard
London EC1A 4JS
Tel: 020 7490 8818
email: info@ukcarers.org
http://www.carersnorth.demon.co.uk

## Counsel and Care (advice and help for older people)
Twyman House
16 Bonny Street
London NW1 9PG
Tel: 020 7485 1550
email: advice@counselandcare.org.uk
http://www.counselandcare.org.uk

## The Court of Protection
The Public Trust Office (Protection Division)
Stewart House
24 Kingsway
London WC2B 6JX
Tel: 020 7269 7300
email: custserv@publictrust.gov.uk
http://www.publictrust.gov.uk

## CRUSE – Bereavement Care
Cruse House
126 Sheen Road
Richmond
Surrey TW9 1UR
Tel: 0208 940 4818
email: info@crusebereavementcare.org.uk

## Dementia Services Development Centres

Offer service information and development, staff training and practice development. They conduct service- and practice-based research, and provide a database and general information about dementia in a local area.

### Dementia North

Wolfson research centre
Newcastle General Hospital
Westgate Road
Newcastle upon Tyne NE4 6BE
Tel: 0191 273 8811
email: ihe@ncl.ac.uk

### Dementia Voice

Blackberry Hill Hospital
Fishponds
Bristol BS16 2EW
Tel: 0117 975 4863/4882
email: office@dementia.voice.org.
http://www.dementia.org.uk

### Ireland DSDC

St James Hospital
St James Street
Dublin 8
Tel: 00 353 1 453 7941
e-mail director@stjames.ie
http://www.dementia.ie

### North Wales DSDC

Tel: John Keady 01248 383779
email: j.keady@bangor.ac.uk
email: dgde@bangor.ac.uk

### North West DSDC

Dover Street Building
University of Manchester
Oxford Road
Manchester M13 9PL
Tel: 0161 275 2000
email: nwdc@man.ac.uk

### Oxford DSDC

Headington Hill Hall
Oxford Brookes University
Headington
Oxford OX3 OBP
Tel: 01865 484706
email: dementia@brookes.ac.uk
http://www.brookes.ac.uk/dementia

## London DSDC (area within the M25)

Tel: Jo Moriarty 020 7504 9588
email: margotlindsay@ucl.ac.uk
http://www.info.ac.nisw.org.uk

## Midlands DSDC

Dementia Plus
(West Midlands)
Wharstones Resource Center
Wharstones Drive
Wolverhampton
WVH 4PQ
Tel: Kate Read 01902 575056

## South East DSDC

Tel: Duncan Callis 01622.725000 (Area Kent, Surrey, Sussex)
email: dcallis@invicta-tr.sthames.nhs.uk

## South Wales DSDC

Tel: Simon O'Donovan 029 2049 4952
email: sdteam@cdff-tr.thames.nhs.uk

## Stirling

University of Stirling
Stirling FK9 4LA
Tel: 01786 467740
email: m.t.marshall@stir.ac.uk
http://www.stir.ac.uk/dsdc

## Trent DSDC

Division of Psychiatry for the Elderly
Leicester General Hospital
Leicester LE54 1PW
email: jeb1@le.ac.uk

## The Journal of Dementia Care

Hawker Publications
13 Park House
140 Battersea Park Road
London SW11 4NB
Tel: 020 7720 2108
email: hawker@hawkerpubs.demon.co.uk
http://www.careinfo.org

## LawNet Ltd (Legal Services)
Ince House
60 Kenilworth Road
Leamington Spa CV32 6JY
Tel: 01926 886990
e-mail: lawnetadmin@lawnet.co.uk
http://www.lawnet.co.uk

## Relate
Herbert Gray College
Little Church Street
Rugby
Warwickshire CV21 3AP
Tel: 01788 573241/560811
email: enquiries@national.relate.org.uk
http://www.relate.org.uk

## Winged Fellowship Trust (holidays for disabled people)
Angel House
20/32 Road
London N1 9XD
Tel: 020 7833 2594
email: admin@wft.org.uk
http://www.wft.org.uk

# References

Alzheimer's Society *Facts and Figures about Dementia.*

Alzheimer's Society – Information Section (2000) (Personal communication.)

Public Affairs Section (2000) (Personal communication.)

Audit Commission (1998) Caring about Carers. Report of the National Stretgy for Carers. Available at http//:www.carers.gov.uk

Audit Commission (2000) *Forget Me Not: Mental Health Services for Older People.* London: HMSO.

Baragwanath, A. (1997) 'Bounce and balance: A team approach to risk management for people with dementia living at home.' In M. Marshall (ed) *State of the Art in Dementia Care.* Centre for Policy on Ageing.

Barclay Report (1982) *Social Workers – Their Roles and Tasks.* London: National Institute of Social Work.

Bowlby, J. (1969) *Attachment and Loss. Vol. 1: Attachment.* London: The Hogarth Press.

Bradford Dementia Group with Kitwood, T. (1997) *Evaluation Dementia Care: the DMC method.* 7th ed. Bradford: Bradford Dementia Group.

Brayne, C. and Ames, D. (1998) 'The epidemiology of mental disorders in old age.' In B. Gearing, M. Johnson and T. Heller (eds) *Mental Health Problems in Old Age.* Chichester: John Wiley Open University.

Brayne, H. and Martin, G. (1990) *Law for Social Workers.* 2nd ed. London: Blackstone Press Ltd.

Bretherton, I. (1995) 'The origins of attachment theory - John Bowlby and Mary Ainsworth.' In Golburg, S. Muir R. and Kerr J. (eds) Attachment Theory: Social Developmental and Clinical Perspectives. New Jersey: The Analytic Press.

Errollyn, B. (1998) 'Holding on to the story: Older people, narrative and dementia.' In Roberts and Holmes (eds) *Healing Stories.* Oxford: Oxford University Press.

Cayton, H. (1997) 'The art of the state: Public policy in dementia care.' In M. Marshall, (ed) *State of the Art in Dementia Care.* London: Centre for Policy on Ageing.

Chapman, A. and Marshall, M. (eds.) (1993) Dementia – New Skills for Social Workers. London: Jessica Kingsley Publishers.

Connolly, J. (1997) 'The hospital.' In *The Blackwell Companion to Social Work.* Oxford: Blackwell Publishers.

Dalley, G. (1996) *Ideologies of Caring – Rethinking Community and Collectivism.* London: Macmillan Press Centre for Policy on Ageing.

Dalrymple, J. and Burke, B. (1995) *Anti-oppressive Practice. Social Care and the Law.* Buckingham: Open University Press.

Department of Health (1998) *Modernising Social Services.* National Priorities Guidance 1999/00-2001/2. London: HMSO.

Department of Health (2000) *Shaping the Future NHS: Long-term Planning for Hospitals and Related Services.* London: Department of Health

Evans, D. (1997) 'Demonstrating competence in social work.' In M. Davies (ed) *The Blackwell Companion to Social Work.* Oxford: Blackwell Publishers.

Goldburg, S., Muir, R. and Kerr, J. (eds) (1995) *Attachment Theory: Social Development and clinical Perspective.* New Jersey: The Analytic Press.

Goldsmith, M. (1997) 'Hearing the voice of people with dementia.' In M. Marshall (ed) *State of the Art in Dementia Care.* London: Centre for Policy on Ageing.

Goodchild, C. (1999) 'Speaking up: Advocacy for people with dementia.' *Journal of Dementia Care* Nov/Dec,19–20.

Haight, B. (1998) 'Use of the life review/life story books in families.' In P. Schweizer (ed) Reminiscence in Dementia Care London: Age Exchange.

Hopker, S. (1999) *Drug Treatments and Dementia.* Bradford Dementia Group Good Practice Guides. London: Jessica Kingsley Publishers.

Jordan, B. (1997) 'Social work and society.' In M. Davies (ed) *The Blackwell Companion to Social Work.* Oxford: Blackwell Publishers.

Keady, J. (1997) 'Maintaining involvement: A meta-concept to describe the dynamics of dementia.' In Marshall, M. (ed) *State of the Art in Dementia Care.* London: Centre for Policy on Ageing.

Killeen, J. (1996) *Advocacy and Dementia*. Edinburgh: Alzheimer Scotland – Action on Dementia.

Killick, J. (1997) *You are Words*. London: Hawker Publications.

Kings Fund (2000) *Report on Kings Fund Seminar on The Health Care needs of Older People*. The Kings Fund.

Kitwood, T. (1997) *Dementia Reconsidered*. Buckingham: Open University Press.

Kitwood, T. and Benson, S. (1995) *The New Culture of Dementia Care. Journal of Dementia Care* Bradford Dementia Group.

LeNavenec, C. (1997) 'Understanding the social context of families experiencing dementia.' In Miesen, B. and Jones, G. (eds) *Care Giving in Dementia Vol. 2*. London: Routledge.

Levin, E. Moriarty J. and Gorbach P. (1994) *Better for the Break*. London: HMSO.

Levin and Webb (1997) 'Social work and community care: Changing roles and tasks.' *Journal of Dementia Care* Sept/Oct.

Lord Chancellor's Office (1997a) *Making Decision*. London: HMSO.

Lord Chancellor's Office (1997b) *Who Decides? Making Decisions on behalf of Mentally Incapacitated Adults*. London: The Stationary Office.

*Managers' and Practitioners' Guide to Care Management and Assessment* (1993). HMSO.

McWalter, G. (1997) 'What do we mean when we talk about assessment?' In M. Marshall (ed) *State of the Art in Dementia Care*. London: Centre for Policy on Ageing.

Miesen, B. (1997) 'Awareness in dementia patients and family grieving. A practical perspective.' In Miesen, B. and Jones, G. (eds) *Care Giving in Dementia*. Vol. 2. London: Routledge.

Moriarty, J. and Webb, S. (1997) *An Evaluation of Community Cares Arrangements Older People with Dementia*. London: National Institute of Social Work.

Office for National Statistics (1998) *Informal Carers*. London: The stationary Office.

Patel, N. and Mirza, N. (2000a) 'Care for ethnic minorities: The professionals' view.' *The Journal of Dementia Care* Jan/Feb, 26-28.

Patel, N. and Mirza, N. (2000b) *Dementia Matters – Ethnic Concerns: The Project*. London: Policy Research Institute on Ageing and Ethnicity.

Payne, M. (1991) *Modern Social Work Theory: A Critical Introduction*. London: Macmillan Press.

Pearson, G. (1975) *The Deviant Imagination: Psychiatry, Social Work and Social Change*. London: Macmillan.

Petch, A.(1997) 'Community Care.' In M. Davies (ed) *The Blackwell Companion to Social Work*. Oxford: Blackwell Publishers.

Phair, L. (1997) 'Elder abuse and dementia: Moving forward.' In M. Marshall (ed) *State of the Art in Dementia Care*. London: Centre for the Policy on Ageing.

Pritchard, J. (1992) *The Abuse of Elderly People*. London: Jessica Kingsley.

*Reform of the Mental Health Act 1983*. Government consultation paper (1999). Stationary Office.

Roper-Hall, A. (1993) 'Developing family therapy services with older adults.' In J. Carpenter and A. Treacher (eds) *Using Family Therapy in the 90s*. Oxford: Blackwell.

Schweitzer, P. (ed) (1998) *Reminiscence in Dementia Care*. Age Exchange.

Seed, P. and Kaye, G. (1994) *Handbook for Assessing and Managing Care in the Community*. London: Jessica Kingsley Publishers.

Shamy, E. (1997) *More than Body, Brain and Breath. A Guide to Spiritual Care for People with Alzheimer's Disease*. New Zealand: Colcom Press.

Sherlock, J. and Gardner, I. (1993) 'Systemic family interventions in dementia.' In Chapman, A. and Marshall, M. (eds) *Dementia – New Skills for Social Workers*. London: Jessica Kingsley Publishers.

Slater, R. and Gearing, B. (1998) 'Attitudes, stereotypes and prejudice about ageing.' In B. Gearing, M. Johnson and T. Heller (eds) *Mental Health Problems in Old Age*. Chichester: John Wiley Open University Press.

Social Services Inspectorate (1990) *Training for Community Care: A Strategy*.

Sutherland, S. (1999) With Respect to Old Age: Long Term care - Rights and Responsibilities. Report by the Royal Commission on Long-term Care. London: The Stationary Office.

Thompson, N. (1993) *Anti-discriminatory Practice*. (BASW series on Practical Social Work.) London: Macmillan Press.

Tibbs, M. A. (1996) 'Amos – a self lost and found.' *Journal of Dementia Care* March/April, 20-21.

Utting, W. (1997) 'A view from central government.' In M. Davies (ed) *The Blackwell Companion to Social Work*. Blackwell Publishers.

Ward, R. (2000) 'Waiting to be heard – dementia and the gay community.' *Journal of Dementia Care*. May/June, 24-25.

White, J. (1997) 'Family therapy.' In M. Davies (ed) *The Blackwell Companion to Social Work*. Oxford: Blackwell Publishers.

# Subject Index

Access to Personal Files Act (1987) 58
acute hospital care 28–31
Admiral Nurse Scheme 157
admission to hospital 28
advocacy 85, 105–6
age 136–8, 154–5
ageing population 13, 56, 63, 146, 150
ageism 56, 88, 154
AIDS-related dementia 138
Alzheimer Europe 34
Alzheimer Scotland – Action on Dementia 15,
    34
Alzheimer's disease 20, 36, 129, 138, 152–3
Alzheimer's Disease International 35
Alzheimer's self-help movement 34–5
Alzheimer's Society 15, 23, 34, 37, 147, 157
    Younger Person Project 138
anti-discriminatory practice 110–11
'anticipatory grieving' 36
appointees 162
Aricept 138
assessment 16, 70–4, 94
    autonomy vs. need for help 72–3
    detention under Section Two 49
    in hospital 28–9
    making contact 70–2
    need for emotional support 73–4
    need for qualitative information 159
    needs-led 18
    time taken 73
    where to conduct 72
attachment theory 96, 112–16, 122

Barclay Report 40, 41, 42–4, 52, 57, 64
Benefits Agency 136, 162
bereavement 36–7
body language, cultural differences 128
Bradford Dementia Group 60, 66

care in the community *see* community care
care management model
    central tasks 51–2
    shortcomings for work with dementia
      119–21, 151–2
Care Needs Assessment Pack (CarenapD) 74
'Care Needs of Ethnic Older Persons with
    Alzheimer's' (CNEOPSA) project 130
care plans 74–84, 94
    multiple clients 74–6
    need for continuous adjustment 77–9, 155
    refusal by carers 82–3

refusal by people with dementia 79–81
    special needs of people living alone 84
care programme approach 49–50
care vs. control 57–8
carers
    abused 92–3
    accepting the move to long-term care 31–2,
      36
    age 13, 21
    benefits of respite care 23–4, 26–7, 115–16
    bereavement 36–7
    contribution of 144
    emotional needs 107–10
    homosexual and lesbian 139
    need for one-stop shop 156
    person-centred training 104
    refusal to accept help 26, 82–3
    separation anxiety 114–15
    stress at time of diagnosis 20–2
    support groups 22–3, 34–5, 37
Carers Act (Carers and Disabled Children's Bill)
    (2000) 56–7
Carers (Recognition and Services) Act (1995) 55
Carers National 37
*Caring about Carers* (Audit Commission) 27
Central Council for Education and Training in
    Social Work 59
Certificate in Dementia Care 60
child protection 56, 57, 59, 64
Children Act (1948) 40
Chronically Sick and Disabled Persons Act
    (1977) 46, 47–8, 67
citizen advocacy 106
'closing cases' 77, 119, 152, 157
'closing down' 103
clothes, cultural differences 128
cognitive impairment 71, 114, 150
communication 101–2
community care
    Griffiths report 44
    key points 53–4
    need for new model 156–9
    philosophy 52
    points of social work interface 23–7
    policy 53
    Royal Commission seminar 54–7
    vs. 'market welfare' 63
community psychiatric nurses (CPNs) 50, 157,
    160
competence-based training 60
'confabulation' 71
confidentiality vs. protection 58–9
connectedness 103
Continuing Power of Attorney 149
costs of care 26, 53, 121, 150

counselling 42, 43, 100
Court of Protection 148, 149, 163–4
CRUSE 37
cultural difference 123–40

Data Protection Act 58
day care 23–5
death 36–7
dementia
    'disaster view' 13–14
    'new culture' 14–15
Dementia Care Mapping (DCM) 66, 151
*Dementia – New Skills for Social Workers* (Chapman
    and Marshall) 16–17
Dementia Services Development Centres 15
demographic patterns 63 *see also* ageing
    population
denial
    carers 82
    people with dementia 80
depression 69
diagnosis 20–3, 150, 156
Diploma in Social Work (DipSW) 60
disability model 152–3
discharge from hospital 29–31
Down's syndrome 138
dual perspective 123–4

early onset dementia 136–8, 154–5
ecomaps 118
elder abuse 59, 92–4, 95
eligibility criteria 64, 68–9, 120–1, 143–4
emotion 97–111, 122
    needs of the carer 107–10
    needs of the person with dementia 100–6
Enduring Power of Attorney 163
    abuse 93
ethnicity 127–33
Exelon 138

families 11
    conflict around care plans 74–6
    discrimination within 111
    emotions 97–100, 107–9
    ethnic minorities 130–1
    financial decisions 165
    shortcomings of the care management model
        119–21
    systems theory 116–18
    use as interpreters 124
family therapy 116, 117
financial abuse 93
financial affairs 162–5
    sale of family home 97–9, 109
*Forget Me Not* report (Audit Commission) 13,
    21–2, 66, 150–1

frontal lobe dementia 23, 137

General Household Survey of Great Britain
    (1995) 144
General Social Care Council 144
generic vs. specialist training debate 59–60
genograms 118
good practice, dissemination 155–6
GPs 20, 21–2, 28, 50, 54, 62, 86, 121, 150,
    156
'grey power' 56
Griffiths Report 44–5, 51
guardianship 50–1, 147

hazards 90–1
health care professionals 73–4, 127, 136
health/social care
    division 44, 54, 55, 61, 156
    joint working 12, 66, 151
helplines 23, 37, 139
hereditary Alzheimer's disease 137
historical overview 39–45
home care 25, 54
    inspection 65–6
homosexual couples 139
hospital
    acute care 28–31
    'bed blockers' 12, 16, 29
Huntington's chorea 138

identity 103
'integrated care' model 62
'intermediate care' 12, 30

'joined-up' working 12, 62, 156
*Journal of Dementia Care* 15, 101, 106

language 124–7
LawNet Ltd 164
legislation 45–54, 55–7, 66–7
lesbian couples 139
local authorities 61, 62, 64, 65, 66, 89, 92
    legal duties and powers 41, 42, 43–4, 46,
        47–8, 56
    unequal services 143, 144–5
Local Authority Social Services Act (1970) 41–2
long-term care *see* residential care
long-term work 43, 64–5, 119–20, 151, 157–8

*Making Decisions* (Lord Chancellor's Office) 142,
    148–9
market model 61–5
medical model 74, 118, 119, 152–3
medical profession 105, 153
Mental Health Act (1983) 46, 49–51, 67, 148
    reform 147–8
mental health social work 57, 59, 60, 120

*Modernising Health and Social Services: National Priorities Guidance* (Department of Health) 12, 141, 142–3
*Modernising Social Services* (Department of Health) 66
multidisciplinary working 54, 156–7
    professional 'pecking order' 104–5
multiple clients 74–6, 119
'multiple oppression' 110–11

National Assistance Act (1948) 40, 45, 46–7, 67
National Association of Carers, The 37
National Beds Inquiry (Department of Health) 30
National Care Standards Commission 65–6
National Health Service 28, 29, 30
    'new NHS' 11–12
    reduction of long-stay beds 146
National Health Service and Community Care Act (1990) 17, 18, 44, 46, 51–4, 61, 63, 64, 67, 120
National Institute for Social Work 42
National Service Framework for Older People 12–13
National Vocational Qualifications (NVQs) 60
new variant CJD 138
nursing homes
    increase in private places 146
    *see also* residential care

older people, generic factors 68–70
one-stop shops 156

'personal detractions' 102–3
personal space, cultural differences 128
person-centred approach 14–15, 20, 25, 71, 84, 101, 104–5, 127, 135
Pick's disease 23, 137
Policy Research Institute on Ageing and Ethnicity, University of Bradford 130
Poor Law 40
Power of Attorney *see* Continuing Power of Attorney; Enduring Power of Attorney
'preferred pathway' route 60
primary care groups 62
'protection of property' procedure 47
psychologists 158
psychotropic medication 158
purchaser-provider split 17, 53, 62

Receivers 163–4
*Reform of the Mental Health Act* 142, 147–8
regulation
    General Social Care Council (GSCC) 144
    national care standards 65–6

residential care 31–6
    comparatively low cost 55
    consent and deception issues 33, 51
    Dementia Care Mapping 66, 151
    dementia-specific standards 147
    effects of the market 61–2, 63–4
    inspection 65
    making the decision 31–3, 108–9
    patchiness of specialist teams 150
    provision of the National Assistance Act 46
    respite 26–7, 115–16
    Royal Commission report 145–7
    settling in 35
    support for carers 34–5, 36
    unnecessary admission 28–9
respite care
    and attachment behaviour 114–16
    day care 23–5
    in the person's home 25
    persuading the person with dementia 80–1
    residential 26–7, 115–16
risk 84–8, 95
    value of formal assessment 89–91
Rogers, Carl 42
Royal College of Nursing 147
Royal Commission into the Funding of Long-Term Care 145, 158
    seminar (1999) 54–5

'sectioning' 147
Seebohm Report 41–2, 59
self-esteem 25, 103, 104, 131
self-help movement 34–5
separation anxiety 114–15
sexual orientation 139
Short Procedure Orders 164
short-term model *see* long-term work
social class 134–6
social policy 53
social security system 41
sporadic Alzheimer's disease 137
spouses and partners 13
    effects of diagnosis 21
    refusal of help 82
    same-sex 37, 139
'strange situation' experiment 112–13
support groups 22–3, 34–5, 37
systems theory 96, 116–18, 122

theoretical approaches 96, 111–18, 122
training 17, 38, 140
    carers 104
    generic/specialised 41, 59–60, 153–4
    regulation 144

'wandering' 85–6

washing, cultural differences 128
welfare state, creation 40–1
Westminster Advocacy Service for Senior
    Residents (WASSR) 106
*Who decides?* (Lord Chancellor's Office) 149
wills 165
*With Respect to Old Age* (Sutherland) 54, 142,
    145–7

younger people with dementia 23, 56, 136–8,
    154–5

# Author Index

Ainsworth and Wittig 112
Alzheimer's Society – Information Section 11,
    23, 24, 121, 137
Alzheimer's Society – Public Affairs Section 56
Audit Commission 13, 21, 27, 66, 150, 156

Baragwanath, A. 90
Bowlby, J. 112
Brayne, C. and Ames, D. 69
Brayne, H. and Martin, G. 40, 45
Bretherton, I. 113
Bruce 113, 114

Cayton, H. 63, 65
Chapman, A. and Marshall, M. 16–17
Connolly, J. 51–2

Dalley, G. 44
Dalrymple, J. and Burke, B. 123–4
Department of Health 12, 30, 66, 141–2

Evans, D. 60

Goldburg, S., Muir and Kerr 112
Goldsmith, M. 102
Goodchild, C. 106
Gurland et al 69

Haight, B. 35
Hopker, S. 158

Jordan, B. 58

Keady, J. 103
Killeen, J. 105–6
Killick, J. 160
Kings Fund 31
Kitwood, T. 14, 100–1, 102, 152–3

Kitwood, T. and Benson, S. 14–15

LeNavenec, C. 118
Levin, E., Moriarty, J. and Gorbach, P. 13, 23–4,
    26, 27, 114–15
Levin and Webb 154
Lord Chancellor's Office 110, 142, 149

McWalter, G. 74
Miesen, B. 36, 100, 101, 107, 114
Milburn, A. 31
Moriarty, J. and Webb, S. 60

Office for National Statistics 13

Patel, N. and Mirza, N. 127, 130
Payne, M. 42, 57
Pearson, G. 57
Petch, A. 53–4
Phair, L. 93–4
Pritchard, J. 92

Roper-Hall, A. 117–18

Schweitzer, P. 160
Seed, P. and Kaye, G. 52, 53, 63
Shamy, E. 160
Sherlock, J. and Gardner, I. 117
Slater, R. and Gearing, B. 88
Sutherland, S. 54, 142, 145, 158

Thompson, N. 110–11
Tibbs, M. A. 133

Utting, W. 44

Ward, R. 139
White, J. 116, 117